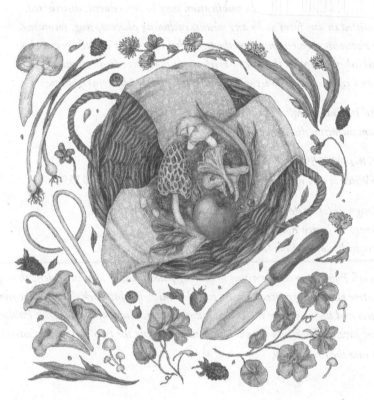

Kitchen Witch

Food, Folklore & Fairy Tale

SARAH ROBINSON

 Womancraft Publishing

Published by Womancraft Publishing, 2022
www.womancraftpublishing.com

ISBN 978-1-910559-69-7
Kitchen Witch is also available in ebook format: ISBN 978-1-910559-68-0

Cover design, interior design and typesetting: lucentword.com
Cover image © Jessica Roux, jessica-roux.com
Illustrations: Bodor Tividar (Shutterstock.com)

Womancraft Publishing is committed to sharing powerful new women's voices, through a collaborative publishing process. We are proud to midwife this work, however the story, the experiences and the words are the author's alone. A percentage of Womancraft Publishing profits are invested back into the environment reforesting the tropics (via TreeSisters) and forward into the community.

Medical disclaimer

I mention within these pages all sorts of thrilling herbs and flowers from ancient texts and old folklore. But please, for the love of goddess, use care if you go out foraging for archangels, whortles and witches' slippers, some of which are best left where they grow. When it comes to gathering herbs and foods from the wild you need to be very careful and know exactly the plant you are seeking, and what you intend to do with it. If in any doubt at all, seek a wise one, be they herbalist, witch, forager or chef.

Also by Sarah Robinson

The Kitchen Witch Companion (with Lucy H. Pearce)
Enchanted Journeys: Guided Meditations for Magical Transformation
Yoga for Witches
Yin Magic: how to be still
The Yoga Witch Cook Book (eBook)
The Yoga Witch Cook Book: Yule Edition (eBook)

Praise for
Kitchen Witch

A fascinating and beautifully crafted book following the history, myths and tales of the Kitchen Witch. Following a trail between legend and modern day working, this makes for a fabulous read.

Rachel Patterson, Kitchen Witch, author of
***Grimoire of a Kitchen Witch* and the *Kitchen Witchcraft* Series**

In Kitchen Witch, Sarah Robinson dishes up an engrossing feast for mind, heart, and spirit. Stewing together lore and legacy and learning, this book will delight you with its blend of commonplace magic, practical enchantment, bits of story, and splashes of curiosity. It reminds us of the power of the arts so often reserved for the realms of women and therefore lost to memory or swept aside as unimportant or mundane.

Kitchen Witch helps us to remember that we come from bread and fire, from resourcefulness and intuition, from tinctures and time, from spiced cider and healing, and from long lines of sweet jellies shining in the sun. We come from the ordinary magic of ordinary lives. In kitchens around the world, we remember.

Molly Remer, MSW, D.Min., priestess, creatrix of #30DaysofGoddess, and author of *Womanrunes*, *Walking with Persephone*, and *Whole and Holy*

This is a thoroughly interesting and important book for all women today, helping us to reclaim our power to interweave our intuitive responses, intentions and healing into the food we create. It is a rich journey into the history and the stories handed down through folklore and folktales, helping us to reach back over the span of time to reconnect with women and women's history, and discover ways to renew our relationship with the land. I shall be buying this for all my women friends this year!

Glennie Kindred, author of *Walking with Trees*,
***Sacred Earth Celebrations* and many more.**

Sarah Robinson continues her engaging explorations of Witchcraft, old and new, through the kitchen door with delicious tidbits, tales and insights to nourish your craft and your spirit.

Phyllis Curott, author of *The Witches' Wisdom Tarot* and *Book of Shadows*

Kitchen Witch is a beautiful and compelling body of work exploring the ordinary, everyday magic in our kitchens: sacred places of connection, listening, healing and cooking.

This invitation to consciously explore what is in our DNA is a marvellous and captivating crossing through the ancient and revered mystical lands of food medicine and magic, ritual and celebration, potions and balms.

From gardens to hedgerows to cauldrons and charms, Sarah Robinson poetically portrays our ancient roots and the calendar of our ancestresses. With the wisdom and skill of the witches who have gone before us, the author draws upon the fields of archaeology, history, mythology, spirituality, fairytale and folklore. These sagesse stories will embed deep into your psyche while the delightful line drawings augment the wisdom of the witches.

Kitchen Witch shows us that our kitchens are holy places of ritual, rhythm, recipes and remembering. Most importantly, we are given permission to live our witchery lives.

Veronika Sophia Robinson, author of *The Mystic Cookfire*, *Love From My Kitchen, I Create My Day;* celebrant and celebrant trainer, and editor of *The Celebrant* magazine

This is a delicious book, which delves into all the corners of the kitchen, and offers insight into how and why we associate certain magic with food.

Alice Tarbuck, author of *A Spell in the Wild*

CONTENTS

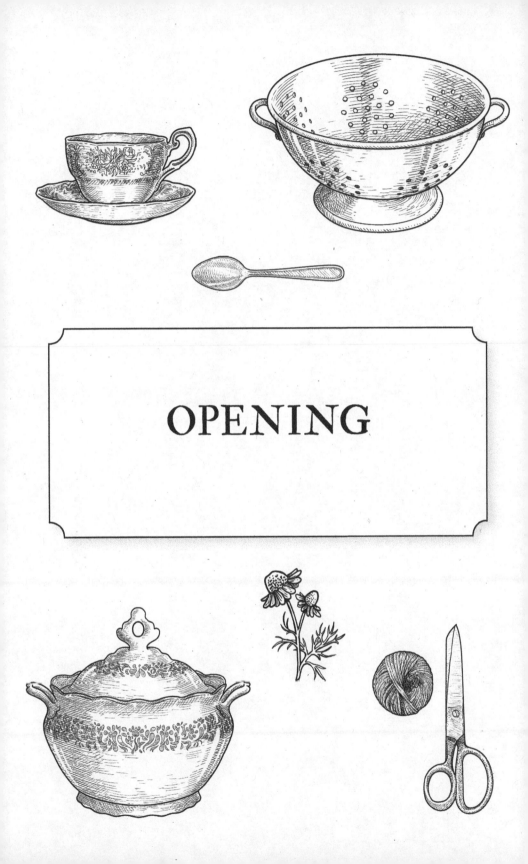

OPENING

A figure stands before a bubbling cauldron, candlelight gleaming through the whorls of steam that rise and dance as liquid is stirred in a spiralling rhythm. What lies inside? Myth and legend may have us guess at a green potion of eyes, limbs and mischief. But every household once owned a cauldron of some kind, so maybe this potion serves a different kind of magic: a nourishing soup to soothe hungry bellies; a stew around which family members will gather; an old jam recipe that conjures memories of someone much missed.

The magic of food and cooking is vast and wide-ranging. It lives in every kitchen, and every person within it. It is the gleam in every story told around the hearth fire, memories brought back to life for a bubbling moment. There is magic woven so intrinsically into the threads of feeding people we love, and the laughter and healing to be found around a dining table, there's nothing quite like it.

This book is just a glimpse into a world of magic in our food: a path scattered with jewel-bright spices, shining fruits and emerald herbs. It is the cacophony of laughter of your dearest friends sat around a table lit by candles. It is a remembering of the tinctures and balms of our ancestors. My dearest hope is to reveal, remind and reconnect you with the magic of food – of which there are so many forms: folklore, superstitions, family recipes, seasonal and celebration feasts. We'll take a journey through magical food history, through some of the history of witches and also of women, often one and the same, their stories snugly intertwined.

The realm of the kitchen can offer such inspiration: practices of folk magic, divination, herbalism, symbolism, sympathetic magic, goddess mythology, potions, balms and feasting foods. And of course, the magic of storytelling. Both in the stories one may tell around a hearth – fairy tales and folklore – and the stories of recipes that may have been handed down through generations.

I am using food and the image of the witch in her kitchen to draw out the contribution of women forgotten through history: their skills and knowledge, their stories. The stories of the Kitchen Witch invite us to reflect upon the history of the witch: how they used vegetables, nuts, flowers and herbs in cooking, charms and remedies and how we might bring forth the legacies of women and wise souls who once sat at the hearth fire, and connect once again to ancient food magic once practiced by all.

ABOUT THIS BOOK

Through the writing of my books on spirituality and mythology, I've worked my way from the east and my role as yoga teacher (in my books *Yoga for Witches* and *Yin Magic*) back home to the spirituality and the folklore of the British Isles and Europe.

Both witchcraft and storytelling are in my blood. All of my collective ancestors – Celtic, Norse and Anglo-Saxon – would have had much knowledge of food, magic, cooking, harvest and the seasons. In fact, every family, village, region and country has its own customs and superstitions when it comes to growing, preparing and consuming food: the stories of food magic are many.

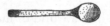

For the most part, we will explore the image and archetype of the Kitchen Witch within Europe, pushing to the outer edges of my homelands. (With the exception of a few stories so special and exciting, I just couldn't bear to leave them out – like Ninkasi, the glorious frothing Sumerian goddess of beer and the rebellions of the chocolate witches of Guatemala.)

I aim to follow threads of the history and practice of food magic from the ancient worlds and first societies to today. My hope is that the threads of these skills, practices and beliefs can inform and strengthen us as we claim the mantle of Kitchen Witch today. Within the kitchen is a world of everyday magic. To seek the magical potential of food is, in itself, a potent ingredient in living an enchanted life. I am drawn to share stories of the women who baked and brewed, who peeled apple skins to spell out messages of love and scattered tea leaves to see the future. My intention with *Kitchen Witch* is to bring these elements further to life for you.

I will be drawing from all kinds of areas: from history, archaeology and anthropology to spiritual, esoteric realms of witchcraft, intuition, and old fairy tales. I'm including in these pages rumours, whispers and stories told to me over a whisky by people whose names I can't remember. This reliance on oral history, stories and domestic wisdom is purposefully chosen. Many women would not have had the means or ability to write down their knowledge: all of their skills would have been passed orally from mother to daughter, from village elder to apprentice. Perhaps some skills that were so unexceptional that our ancestors simply couldn't imagine a world where people no longer knew how to bake bread, or cure meat, treat with herbs or track the sun's progress for the harvest. Many of these domestic practices that were vital for life for so much of our history have been lost – or diminished – by modernity and the dominance of professional history and the written word.

I am looking forward to recounting a few of the stories (imperfectly recorded as they may be) of some of the women tried as witches: words from Alice Duke, Isobel Gowdie and Agnes Sampson. We will also learn more about many goddesses and deities connected with food: Brigid, Walpurga and Lussi (who, as English writer Karl Pearson puts it, may well have "received a slight coat of whitewash from the early Christians" and reappeared as virgins and saints in stories we learned at school) as well as those who, by contrast, were cast into deep shadow – Kerridwen, Medea, and Perchta. We will unravel pagan practices, folk customs, rural superstitions and goddess worship from various cultures that the Church and patriarchal authorities tried to cast out and repress. By piecing together these wisps of history and folklore, we can see a wealth of parallels and identical customs in charms, festivals, prayers and the veneration of saints and goddesses alike and their connections to our daily lives today, through the food we eat and the place we prepare it.

Kitchen Witch is part of my own journey of remembering, recognising, and reviving the fullness of the witch, by bringing to light just some of the stories: the awful and the joyful, the everyday and the exceptional.

No Recipes? Really?

For a book about kitchens and food, you may be surprised to learn – and I'll repeat this now to guide your expectations – *there are no detailed recipes in this book.*

Kitchen Witch is a book of tales tied tightly around food, and perhaps these stories illustrate, in the best way I can, that you don't always need exact recipes (or spells) to make magic. You don't need them to see food's fantastic potential to heal, to see the magical possibilities of the kitchen realm…or to claim your authority as a Kitchen Witch. It is rather the magic, medicine and memory that food and cooking evoke that we will focus on here.

This is not going to be a book of facts, figures and precise measurements, although there are a few strewn about like pomegranate seeds. There are going to be stories in this book that are different from how you know them, there may well be some traditions that are new to you, as well as some that are very familiar, and some I have purposely rewoven.

KITCHEN WITCH:
FOOD, FOLKLORE AND FAIRY TALE

I will begin by laying out my path, just a little, in breadcrumbs to help guide our way.

Let's take a look at each element of the title of this book: *Kitchen Witch: Food, Folklore and Fairy Tale* so that you might see the part they will play in our journey.

KITCHEN WITCH

Kitchen witchcraft is, in essence, the magic of hearth, home and food. And the term enjoys many positive associations. The magical can become part of daily life when the kitchen is considered a sacred space. And for millennia it has been just that.

The kitchen is where we all once gathered, shared knowledge, discovered the secrets and alchemy of plants, created remedies, and became the first healers, nurses, midwives and early physicians. We learned how to nourish and sustain ourselves and families, transferring skills and gaining knowledge. There is forgotten magic in the kitchen as a sacred space.

The Kitchen Witch will be our guide and teacher for this journey. You may be familiar with her already, or perhaps know her by other names. Though not everyone wishes to identify as a witch, the title taps into a sacred lineage of women's knowledge about healing, spiritual practice and the earth.

Many strands of cultural and spiritual heritage were and are carried in skilled hands by women and those who may have called themselves witches. This carrying was done through every craft of home and hearth: spinning, weaving, herb craft, divination, song, prayer, ritual, and the topic I have prioritised, cooking and crafting of food. The Kitchen Witch reminds us all that the ordinary arts of daily life have a magical quality: the alchemy of cooking, the herbal magic in your garden, stories at your own hearth are to be valued and treasured.

On Magic

Magic is ancient. The awareness of an unseen world beyond our day-to-day existence is something all cultures have recognised in some way. Like science and religion, magic can imbue us with a sense of hope, empowerment, and perhaps help us to understand a little better the wider world and universe we inhabit. Magic is also a distinct way of participating in one's life and potentially influencing the direction in which we travel. Through every culture magic has been used to seek and understand the past, present and future, protect from harm and promote wellbeing through connecting to deities or the energy of personal strengths.

Magic is a rich broth of words, images and associations that may dwell beyond (or be hidden from) scientific understanding. It can include crafts, skills, sets of practices that are infinitely malleable, that can be made into art, ceremony, and therapy and is, of course, central to the world of fairy tales and practice of witches, ancient and modern. Magic is alive.

We will explore who the Kitchen Witch is and has been, from the good cook and kindly homemaker, potion maker and sacred hearth-keeper, to witches of gingerbread houses and the poppets that hang from herb strewn rafters for good luck. We will delve deep into the history, archetype, and many incarnations of the Kitchen Witch in the first section.

To follow the path of kitchen witchcraft can be joyful and sumptuous. But, make no mistake, this joy is hard-won. The history of witchcraft is a challenging one to delve into. Amazing rituals and customs lie in foundations of ashes: torture and trials that we can barely imagine now. There has been a battle to get to this place. This is a book of delights, but just like the fairy tales I'll be sharing, there are dark and serious elements, drawn from roots of suffering and despair. From the stories of Persephone to Rapunzel to the modern witch hunts, there are accounts of mistreatment, abuse, imprisonment, and injustice that are undeniably challenging. And much like in fairy tales, there are significant themes of love, loss, desperation, hunger and hate.

We'll be peeking behind the myth to find the many forms and names of the Kitchen Witch throughout time: priestess, cook, alewife, cunning woman, herbalist – all, in their time have connected to and symbolised magic in the kitchen in some way. We'll be seeking out myriad ideas and images of Kitchen Witches and magic workers within food, folklore and fairy tale. I invite you to journey with me as I explore text and history, legends and myths, finding fascinating morsels of who and what the Kitchen Witch really is…

FOOD

From our earliest days as hunter-gatherers, it was women who stoked the first hearth fires, stirred the first pots, brewed the first beer and baked the first bread.

Danielle Prohom Olson from 'Reclaiming the Magical Herstory of Food' for GatherVictoria.com (2017)

To reveal the *herstory* of food is to tell the stories of women's skills and wisdom that have been lost or left out of historical accounts. The stories that *have* endured of women are often in the form of stereotypes: the witch cackling over a cauldron; screeching fishwives; images of troublesome women of questionable reputations – all historical embodiments of that double-edged phrase "well-behaved women seldom make history."[1] Whereas the vital daily work of cooking and nourishing has fallen through the floorboards of history, like crumbs of toast, and the best-remembered tales are often the least flattering: cruel and strongly biased.

Women created many of the processes of cooking, baking, preservation and food storage. This is what Max Dashu, author and academic (and maven of bringing the suppressed histories of women into the light) calls "mother-tech": creations of now-forgotten women, working out of view and without recognition, quietly weaving prayers and magic into the food they created. This is a magic trick of sorts: the inventive power of women's work, and their fantastical transformations within the kitchen. She makes it all appear so ordinary, this conjuring of meals, of turning houses into homes, creating families and to weaving both tales and blankets by the hearth fire. The history of food is the history of women. And magic, hearth and kitchen are all woven together and wrapped up in that too. So some of these pages will explore directly the work and lives of those we called witches, but also of women who practiced other skills.

Long ago, each act of food production, planting, harvesting, preserving, baking, were done as ritual crafts, to the rhythm of women's songs, stories, blessings and prayer. Central to this was an honouring of the Earth Mother, household deities, spirits and ancestors – who in turn were thought to watch over the household, its health and harvest. All across the ancient world, whether they called her Ninkasi, Fornax, Demeter, Hecate, Vesta or Hestia, women have carved the Goddess' sacred symbols onto pots and hearthstones and laid icons at home altars, made offerings to her as they gathered food from the fields and prepared it at the hearth. Like fairy tales, stories of the Goddess can tell us much about the people that created them. But the Goddess and her stories have been hidden and transmuted. Few of us know that we have goddesses to thank for some of our most cherished food customs. For example, the Greek goddess Artemis was honoured with round cakes topped with candles to represent moonlight, and we all now expect sweet treats with flames on at birthdays!

Bread, cakes, fruits and wine were offered up at altars and tables for the Goddess in seeking much needed blessings to ensure health, prosperity and abundance for crops, homes, families and lands. We often forget that our ritual feasts and seasonal celebrations we hold today were once a very serious and significant business: life in centuries past was short, brutal, full of uncertainty, and there was true fear that angering the gods/goddesses would result in disaster.

Years when harvests were poor were called "need years" and required "need foods": nettles, acorns, wild herbs, berries, seaweed... An accumulated ethnobotanical knowledge about foods that could be foraged in hard times like these would be vital for a community. These foods may well have had magical properties – but nourishment and food during times of extreme hunger are magic enough in their own right.

For most of us, either because of having enough food, or because of our disconnection from nature, we no longer see the magic of plants to offer healing, the significance of needfoods when we are starving, or the comfort bought by making offerings to the goddesses of the harvest. Maybe we don't interact with our food so much now that we aren't growing it or preparing it as necessity. It may be that we don't see or notice our food, let alone the magic of it.

On Gender

I do not wish to exclude anyone from these stories, but I do want to tell you some important ones that involve women, and how their stories are relevant to us all. Our journey in this book is going to take us around some heavily gendered ideas, as many accused witches – especially the ones that suffered most during witch trials – *were* women (around 80% of victims of the European witch hunts were women, 90% in the British Isles). Much oppression of women was done under the guise of the witch hunts, and I don't want to lose that fact in the re-telling.

It is important to remember that it was never *just* men versus women or Church versus witches, (some men and church officials actively condemned the witch trials), but they do play a large part in these stories. The story of cooking, like witchcraft, includes many conventionally feminine skills and crafts. And when it came to the alewives, herb-wives, and all of the day-to-day kitchen work, that was a female-dominated affair. I want to acknowledge this historical legacy. We can draw from this reflection of the past and embrace the magic of food moving forward as open and available to all genders.

From the Neolithic to the early modern era, all genders were healers, herbalists, magic-makers and wise ones. Men were accused and killed as witches too.[*] Many of us know that already, but I want to just reiterate it here: all genders suffered. What we see at play is the archetype of the ruler and destroyer seeking to dominate that of the nurturer and nourisher.

Like folklore, passed through generations, we are changing all the time, and hopefully, this is an opportunity to reflect and grow. Now, in the twenty-first century, "witch" is a gender-neutral term. Whatever your gender identity, it is my intention and hope that you'll find some interesting ideas and magical tales here.

---

[*] There is a huge volume of evidence of misogyny on the part of those persecuting witches. Many judges and lawmakers would perpetuate stereotypes by sharing their experiences convicting women in print in so-called 'witch hunting manuals.' Jean Bodin, *Of the Demon-mania of the Sorcerers* (1580); Nicolas Remy, *Demonolatry* (1595) and Pierre de Lancre *On the Inconstancy of Witches* (1612). Female witches already had "one foot in hell" (de Lancre), women are more "susceptible to evil counsels" (Remy). These judge-authors, and others like them were responsible for countless innocent women's deaths both from their books and the sentences they cast.

It is also important to note that there are a few cases (in Iceland, Russia and Normandy, France) where more men than women were found guilty and killed as witches. And a few other places like Finland, Estonia and Latvia that saw closer to even gender splits. However, overall, it seems impossible to deny that women were targeted with extreme bias.

Folklore and superstition, if nothing else, may help us see food in a different way or consider the benefits of a herb or plant. Cooking was, and can be, a source of empowerment, a living tradition, connecting us back to ourselves and our ancestors. And we can be empowered in our role as provider. But the herstory of food is complicated. There have been significant periods when women have felt oppressed, defined by their place in the kitchen and by food: trapped and 'chained to the kitchen sink.' Food has also been a central player in the cultural control of women's bodies, the perpetual hell-cycle that is diet culture, being told what and how we should eat.

Today the professional world of cooking is dominated by men (studies over the last three years in the UK and USA have found that less than a quarter of professional chefs are women) which I am not bemoaning but offering up as a point of reflection as to where masculine energy sometimes dominates. And as reminder that as with the healing arts, when cooking and brewing left the domestic sphere and became places where significant money and status could be earned, they swiftly became governed by specialised guilds that excluded women.

Nonetheless, food is still deeply entwined with the feminine.

Food-lore and food-ways have not always been considered a serious area of study. Because, for so long, food was the realm of the housewife, cook and crone, this mundane, domestic creation of nourishment and healing was often overlooked or dismissed. But historians, anthropologists and folklorists do now recognise the role of food as an integral part of daily life as well as ritual and ceremony, customs, belief and superstition.

Food memories involve the most primal, nonverbal areas of the brain. We can have strong emotional reactions when a food awakens deep unconscious memories, connections with powerful layers of food memory, like bridges to our own personal history. The taste, smell, and texture of food can be extraordinarily evocative, bringing back memories not just of eating a food itself, but also of place, setting and the emotions of that moment. The act of cooking can reawaken memories and create new ones, transporting us through time, boundary and place. It is ancient, yet brand-new, each time we step into the kitchen with fresh ingredients and intentions.

I hope to illuminate food as an integral element of celebrating the natural year and the cycle of life, so that we can forge a deeper, more meaningful connection to the ingredients and cooking techniques that we use to nourish ourselves. In reclaiming our lost food traditions, we may once more find the magic of making and sharing food. Acknowledging the women that were a huge part of food magic and the very heart of early food history is part of that reclaiming.

FOLKLORE

Folklore is a community-held and created knowledge of customs and celebrations intertwined with daily life, beliefs and practices that are informally learned and passed on through stories, songs, recipes, remedies, gossip and superstitions through family lines and social circles. Folklore is a vessel for essential communal knowledge: knowledge that was once vital to survival.

Exploring regional superstitions and folklore help us to understand the history and culture of a place and its people, their fears, hopes and beliefs, and reflect how people reacted to life's uncertainties. Both food and the stories involving food, give us a sense of a culture, a time and place, telling us something about the people who prepared it, ate it, and offered it up in ceremony. Often folklore can seem quaint, strange, a distant old-fashioned idea of times gone by, but folklore is still with us, constantly changing and growing. Our understanding of folk practices and superstition may have changed and developed, but they are still powerful practices.

Folklore reminds us of and connects us to heritage, community, time and tradition. And we see new rituals and practices emerging all the time, gathering their own stories that will, in time become their own lore of practices and celebrations that are part of seeing in new eras or seasons. Like gifting chocolate at Easter, certain festive parades, pumpkins signalling a home offering candy, new customs for weddings and baby showers, birthdays, and bank holidays, 'urban legends' we heard in our childhood that become folktales of the county, myths around the internet and technology. Some are new variations on old themes and some are new customs, new ways to celebrate and remember what is important.

With the rise of digital media, television and the internet, it may feel that spoken stories, myths and folklore tales have become less relevant. But perhaps it's simply that we are seeing them in new forms: blockbuster films using deities from Norse mythology, fairy-tale inspired fiction, computer games and music albums inspired by folklore. One might question the importance of these old stories, but they are everywhere if we seek to find them. We may no longer seek them to tell us how the world came into creation, but they are rich in the beliefs and values of our ancestors.

Fairy Tale

Fairy tales are a part of folklore, but tend to feature more fantastical ideas about people, fairies, animals, or objects who have magical powers. In contrast, folk tales are the traditional beliefs and practices of a culture passed down orally through stories. Both fairy tales and folk tales can be instructive: they might leave the reader with a lesson or warning. Their deeper meaning ultimately brings longevity, as lessons learned from shared stories are passed among cultures and generations. Folk tales can derive in part, from real-life phenomena, from the seemingly magical: will o' the-wisps and fairy circles of mushrooms, to the devastating: illness and crops failing.

Fairy tales are usually not completely literal in their plots and messages, unlike folklore which at one point people (or at least some people) believed to hold some truth. They were never written as 'true' tales. There is a quote attributed to Albert Camus that sums it up nicely: "Fiction is the lie through which we tell the truth." Fairy tales are a fiction but within them lie many truths, for example, what one may do in case of extreme fear or hunger. Others make very little logical sense, yet still they endured, to scare or entertain. Life is perhaps every bit as strange, wonderful, horrifying, and unbelievable as the fairy tales so there is wisdom within them, and sometimes truth as well.

She's away with the fairies...

With her publication *Fairy Tales (Les Contes des Fées)* in 1697, Madame d'Aulnoy (Marie-Catherine Le Jumel de Barneville, Baroness d'Aulnoy) coined the term "fairy tale". She also popularised some very well-known stories and motifs (such as coaches made of pumpkins) which we recognise today, an accolade I feel she deserves to be better known for. I am purposely sharing her work and words into this book, deservedly side by side with Perrault, Grimm, and Christian Anderson, male authors with whom we are all more familiar.

Fairy tales were told for entertainment, often for adults as well as children. Some of the first and most well-known printed collections of fairy tales – *Tales and Stories of the Past with Morals* (or *Tales of Mother Goose*) by Charles Perrault (1697), *Fairy Tales* by Marie-Catherine d'Aulnoy (1697), *Children's and Household Tales* by Jacob and Wilhelm Grimm (1812) and *Tales Told for Children* by Hans Christian Anderson (1835) – indicate strongly in the titles that these tales are intended to be told to children. They all, however, feature infanticide, abuse, cannibalism, dismemberment, and disembowelment. Though one might argue that many kids love to hear such gruesome tales, we are often told the 'nicer' versions in the present day (such as via the work of Disney), and some more frightening folk tales may be 'softened' to create more whimsical fairy tales. But the stories also introduce children to very important ideas of what cruelty and hatred may lead someone to do, as well as the virtues of kindness, diligence and honesty and the reward inherent in those. These elements make fairy tales particularly valuable for children (and us all). There is often a very clear-cut 'goodie' and 'baddie,' and morals that support lessons we hold for the rest of our lives: the importance of finding your happily ever after; kissing a few frogs before you find a prince; not taking food from strangers; lying has consequences and hard work will be rewarded. They can also give form and language to fears, which can help children understand and articulate real-life troubles and stressors. As adults, we may find some of these stories comforting as familiar tales or inspiring as we explore them again, finding new meaning and ways through which we can explore emotions, life events and uncertainty.

The stories and lessons within fairy tales are often blends of elements of classic legends and ancient mythology, recounted over generations, evolving into amalgamations of morality tales with the same features: the witch in the forest; the hero's quest; battles of good versus evil.

The whispers of truth within these tales often spoke to real-life struggles, and here folklore, history and fairy tale meet: just as witches existed in all three spheres, so did cruel parents, starving children, strangers in woods… This would have made them more fascinating and relevant to the lives of those reading and telling the tales and aided their longevity.

We love to separate and categorize. But fairy tales, superstition and folktales are fascinating (amongst many other reasons) because they work in a kind of liminal space. The folklore and superstitions surrounding food in these stories are on a spectrum: will salt thrown over your shoulder blind the devil that sits there? Probably not. Will a potion of herbs such as mint or chamomile have a physiological effect on your body? Yes, absolutely. Finding treasure within a walnut – well, sort of, although it won't be a ball gown in there! Seeing messages or the future in coffee, to some skilled people, yes, that's a reality, and cauldrons *are* a place where magic can be brewed, whether that be the brew of the alewives or housewives, the knowledge inspired by deities or the handed-down knowledge of simple herbal remedies. There's magic to be found if you look carefully enough…

Whose Stories?

I did not create the fairy tales I will share in this book, of Hansel and Gretel, Cinderella, Rapunzel, the witch in her egg boat and the laughing bean who splits her sides. They are stories that have travelled through centuries and countless cultures. I have delighted in uncovering them in old books and then retelling them.

When I repeat these stories, it is with humility and respect – these are not my stories, but for this moment, in this place I am their carrier, just as anyone who retells them is. These are not my stories: these are *our* stories, stories that travel, stories that endure.

Folk tales are owned by no one, which is part of what makes them so special. They can be shared, retold, studied by anyone who wishes to do so, who sees their value and their entertaining wisdom. But treating them with openness on their origins as best I know them is how I try and avoid appropriation and seek to be mindful and respectful with these precious words and cultural heritage.

Welcome

So, welcome all! I have stories of sumptuous food to share, tales to tell, and ideas to whisper. There is herstory and history of the cauldron, kitchen and hearth fire to revive. Together we will remember old ways, past stories of times gone by and the infinite possibilities within the alchemy of cooking. We will rediscover the magic of food and bringing people and words together – in love and celebration, healing, memory and myth.

Magic, like witch, means different things to different people. It is something I think we need now more than ever before. I said it myself in my last book, *Yin Magic*, "Magic teaches us that things that seem to be impossible can become possible. Things that have become separated, blocked or broken, like people and energy, can be re-joined. We can find the light, find space, and the empty cauldrons can be refilled with time and love."

Perhaps you consider yourself a witch…or seek to become one. Maybe you are interested in the stories of the kitchen, the cauldron and craft, ancient deities, folklore, superstitions and the history of food. The archetype of the witch can weave together strands of these pasts, the present, and the future, to become a catalyst for change and how we approach our relationship to food, feasting, and magic.

These stories, I hope, will bring you closer to the foods you eat, or perhaps closer to finding delight in the daily process of creating food for yourself and others. I have tried to organise these amazing tales, superstitions, magical whisperings as best I can into sections: The Kitchen Witch in History and Archetype; Food in Folklore; Food for Magic and Healing, and Food for Celebration. But there will be many blurred edges and crossovers. For example, I have delighted in sharing, with the help of talented brujas, the history and magic of coffee in the Food Magic section, but you'll also find folktales that feature coffee as a supplier of portents and a catalyst for change in the Folklore section. The same with nuts: you'll find them in Food Magic, Food in Folklore and Food for Celebration sections, as we weave through the stories of nuts in fairy tales as purveyors of treasures, but also the real-life practices and traditions of Nut-Crack Night. So, like all good fairy tales, as we get lost in the forest of stories, you may discover things not quite where you expect them!

Together we'll venture out around the homestead, community, and natural world. We will forage and gather together. But we'll always come back to the kitchen, and through food, seek to find our way back 'home'.

So, let's head into the kitchen, the witch is waiting…

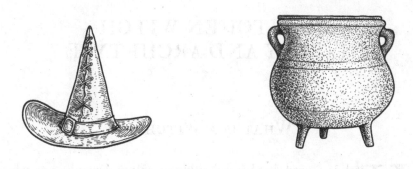

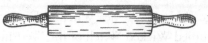

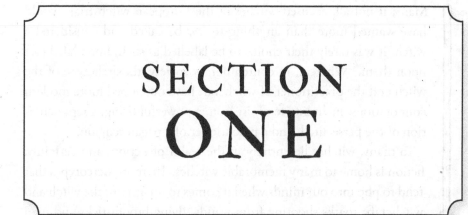

SECTION
ONE

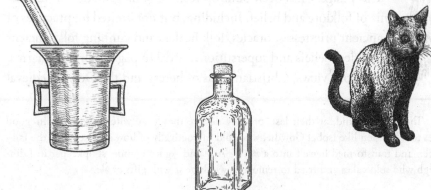

THE KITCHEN WITCH –
HISTORY AND ARCHETYPE

What is a Witch?

Witch is a word that has polarising meanings depending on where you are and who is wielding the word, ranging from proudly claimed and celebrated title, to insult or even death sentence. Historically, a witch was someone who used magic, also called witchcraft. To some, this might mean magic for any purpose, where 'good magic' was acceptable; for others, all magic was considered dangerous or harmful. Many, if not all, accused witches of the European witch trials would have wanted more than anything to *not* be called and considered a witch: it was rarely their choice to be labelled as such, but a label cast upon them.[*] Whereas, in contemporary society, the archetype of the witch and the practitioner of witchcraft have developed more modern connotations, including feminist icon, a powerful being, a representation of the persecuted, and a practitioner of a pagan religion.

To many, witches lie entirely in the realm of fiction, and certainly, fiction is home to many memorable witches. There are stereotypes that tend to pop into our minds when it comes to imagery of the witch and witchcraft: sparks shooting from wands, flying broomsticks and men turned into frogs. Folklore and literature from ancient times to the modern day are peopled with diverse witches: most of us can easily recall the image of Ursula the Sea Witch in Disney's *Little Mermaid* or the green skinned Wicked Witch of the West in *The Wizard of Oz*.

This imagery has been built up from an amalgamation of millennia of folklore and belief. Including, but not limited to: practices of ancient priestesses, oracles, folk healers and cunning folk, ancient goddess beliefs and superstitions, ritual in pagan Europe, charms, religious views, Christian ideas of heresy and the Devil, medieval

---

[*] Though some did, at their last, proudly declare they were witches and flippin' good ones too! Women like Isobel Gowdie, who told so poetically of how she met with the fairy queen and transformed herself into a *mickle hare* and Agnes Fynnie, shopkeeper in Edinburgh who sold cakes and tried to remove bewitchment with gifts of ale.

and early modern practice of ceremonial magic and alchemy. All these influences have come together to create a very formidable and complex construct.

Meeting Baba Yaga

When it comes to witches in folklore and fairy tale, few can compare with the mother/crone/hag figure of Baba Yaga. Many witches in stories and fairy tales don't even get the honour of a name: they are simply an archetypal/stereotyped witch figure. By contrast, Baba Yaga is a fierce force of magic, who, when approached with caution, can help or destroy.

Tales of Baba Yaga appear in folktales of Russia, Ukraine, Poland and Belarus. In various Eastern European languages, Baba may mean elderly woman, grandmother, midwife, sorceress or fortune teller, and Yaga connects to words "ag/aga" for cauldron and fire, so she could certainly be called a Kitchen Witch.

It was the Babas – both the fictional and real-life – who gathered the wild herbs, tended the beehives, ground grain, baked in ovens, and advised the community on rituals of healing, birthing and dying. Tales of Baba Yaga, like similar stories in other countries, may well have played a part in demonising the old village wise women and healers: the fearful and ignorant accused these people of being witches and using their powers for evil.

In Russian lore, Baba Yaga flies across the sky in a mortar and pestle, with a broom made of silver birch to sweep away any trace of her path. Sometimes, we see her flying in a cauldron too, utilising everyday kitchen tools that were also tools for medicine and magic.

The Baba Yaga story character lives deep in the forest, representing, perhaps, the more wild, untamed and unpredictable forces of nature and the dark winter seasons. Yet she could also be generous, kind, and compassionate. Like many old witches of folklore, her kitchen was often filled with edible riches (sometimes gathered by malevolent means). In many stories, she offers the hero or heroine something to eat and/or to drink or asks for food herself. Anyone who seeks her advice must be prepared for danger because a risky task will be required of them to gain Baba Yaga's help. Those approaching her for assistance must have a purity of heart and spirit and treat her with respect. Depending on the story, Baba Yaga may be helpful...or eat you and add your bones to her garden fence – she's tricksy like that!

The witch in a story can represent evil, justice, magical power, jealousy and the persecuted innocent. And it's often hard to prise apart the truth, not least because witches are rarely just one thing: not just a character of good or bad, but one that can both help and hinder, offer both blessings and fury. And perhaps this is precisely why we are so captivated by the image of the witch, because, in fable and tale, they are a more complex character than the handsome prince, the demure princess, the benevolent king: the witch is many things.

Witch – Myth and Reality

The myth of the witch, the one whose image we see in fairy tales, is different from the evil women that the Church and witch hunters spoke of. And she is very different again from the witch of 'the real world.' But they all live under this banner of the name Witch. So, we will meet her (and his, and their) many different faces, archetypes and incarnations, all of which can teach us something, about fear, bias, stereotype, but also the longevity of these superstitions and images and the value of these stories. This is not always an easy task: sifting through what is truth and what is fiction, what we know, what we assume, and what has been lost to time.

Witches of the Ancient World

The persecution of witches was not unique to the periods of Europe's witch trials (though this time did see some peaks in numbers). It actually began to emerge in the ancient world.

Magic in ancient Egypt and Mesopotamia was not feared, although using spells to harm others still came with punishments. It is in ancient Greece and Rome that we see the fog of fear around witchcraft begin to appear around rural and pagan traditions, a fear that would in time see witchcraft painted as a sin and a crime.

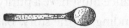

The witch serves various roles in Greek and Roman imagination:[*] she represents popular fears and fantasies either as a magical helper or as a destructive force. So, although real women of these ancient Greco-Roman civilisations could make a living by offering healing, love potions, protection spells and curses, helping in daily matters as well as serving as a connection to the divine and/or spirit world, being known for doing so was dangerous, and practitioners were always at risk of being accused by authorities or unsatisfied clients.

When illness swept through Rome around 331 BCE, almost two hundred women were executed as witches, thought to be responsible for poisoning the population.[2] And one of the most detailed accounts of a witchcraft trial in Greece is the story of Theoris of Lemnos, a folk healer who was executed along with her children supposedly for casting incantations and using potions, in around 338 BCE. The witch had well and truly moved from the realm of myth into the day-to-day lives and fears of both Greeks and Romans.

The crime of sorcery in Roman law was punishable by death, but petitions to deities like offerings at altars and curse tablets were commonplace, so magic work and deity worship were still part of day-to-day practice. It was poisons and love potions which may cause someone to act against their will, that seemed to concern authorities the most, along with powerful women...

A woman in a position of control was a troubling notion to many in the classical era, and the the possibility of a woman overpowering a man with mystical powers or potions was seen as a serious problem. Myths gave voice to primal patriarchal fears of powerful women seeking retribution, embodied in the mythic Furies, three Greek goddesses of vengeance who punished men for their crimes, from their Underworld home they ascended to earth to pursue the wicked. Imagery such as snaked hair and bat wings added the idea of them being terrifying creatures.

You might recognize the names such as Circe, Medea and Hecate from classical myth and literature – these fictional sorceresses (who we shall meet a little later) inhabited the margins of society, symbolizing and personifying peripheries, edges and boundaries. These witches made a big impression and these ancient stereotypes have persisted, with their characterisations still acting as 'templates' for the portrayal of witches today.

---

[*]   The Classical eras of Ancient Greece (800/1000 BCE to 323 BCE) and Ancient Rome (753 BCE to 476 CE) were close both in time and geographically, so they often connect and overlap when it comes to cultural ideas and myths, and are sometimes grouped together as the Greco-Roman world, as period of cultural history.

European Witch Hunts

During the witch hunts of Europe, we see ceremony and celebration warped and twisted by those who wanted an elaborate evil, a scapegoat to strike fear into the heart of people in order to ensure adherence to mainstream religious belief. These myths and superstitions have woven into, and around, the real world, affecting the stories of real witches and real women. There is a vast range of contrasting views about who the persecuted European witches were. We don't, and can't, know the full story. Even how many died during the witch hunts is a guess. At present, the figure from many scholars and historians ranges from 60,000 at the lower end and up toward 100,000 to 200,000 (which is a wide scope to say the least).[*] However, a huge number of variables just aren't accounted for: unofficial means of "justice," persecution outside of the vague witch hunt date brackets from the end of the Middle Ages into the early modern era – (1400-1800), victims dying awaiting trial, trials outside of Europe and other events that saw witches burnt such as the Inquisition, make it very hard to pin anything down with any certainty.

A Note on the Nine Million...

I know many readers may have higher numbers in mind when it comes to numbers of victims of the witch-hunts, as the highest estimates run up into the millions. I turned to the work of Professor Ronald Hutton, who mentions how we got the figure of nine million in *Witches, Druids and King Arthur*. He refers to German historian Gottfried Christian Voigt who based his work on the number of witches killed in his hometown (Germany had the highest death toll during the witch hunts *by far*, way above anywhere else in Europe) and he took this number and created an average assuming every other European city had done the same over a period of a thousand years or so. Thus, he reported in

---

[*]   Drawn from various estimates from historians and scholars in the field – the likes of Ronald Hutton, Max Dashu, Anne L. Barstow, Owen Davies, and Brian Levack. All have their own estimates, some reflections on the estimates of others, so this is an amalgam of some of those numbers. I believe, at the very least, we can agree they are appalling and significant numbers.

an article in 1784 *"Etwas über die Hexenprozesse in Deutschland"* ("A few words about witch trials in Germany"), his estimate of the figure of 9,442,994 executions between 600 and 1700 CE. This is a much larger timeframe than many historians use, but I think wholly appropriate, as we know people have been persecuted for malefic magic centuries before and after just the 'peak' of the witch hunts.

Over time, notable folks accepted and repeated Voigt's number, such as Matilda Joslyn Gage, In *Woman, Church and State* (1893), Andrea Dworkin in *Women-Hating* (1974) and in the 1990 witch documentary *The Burning Times*. It is unlikely that historians will ever be able to settle on a figure for the death toll of the European witch hunts, let alone all witch hunts worldwide. I personally think if we could somehow know every soul who has died from being accused a witch – yes, I think that would be in the millions, so I don't consider the claim unreasonable, but if you were studying just the European early modern witch trials, perhaps that would be closer to the tens or hundreds of thousands.

This mass slaughter of people – whether they were witches or not – was a destruction not only of human life and community – parents, children, friends and lovers – but also skills and knowledge: of medicinal plants, wild foods and where to find them, spells and charms, midwifery skills, recipes passed down through generations. Like the burning of the lost libraries of Alexandria, this was a burning of knowledge, systematic cultural desecration. All the more reason to treasure and reconnect to accounts, stories and folklore.

We understand better now that those accused of witchcraft *were* the victims of (amongst other variables) a controlling Church, seekers of scapegoats, political motives and/or jealous neighbours, angry and fearful communities. But also, that some of the accused were people carrying on traditions of healing, herbalism, divination and spirituality from pre-Christian eras. Communing with the spirit of the lands and ancestors, fairies and other nature spirits and remnants from a distant past – a past that would come to be seen as threatening to new world views that did not encourage such use of intuition, dreams and visions.

Anything could be, and often was, blamed on the Devil and his hand-maidens: witches. Many of these "quarrelsome dames" as they were referred to in some of the Scottish witch trials, considered themselves Christian, but also believed in magic, and charms, perhaps offering up these skills to earn a little money – and were probably bewildered by suggestions that they were cavorting with demons. They, like everyone else, were simply trying to survive, all the harder in a past world often filled with famine and illness.

There is (and always will be) much debate around how many of those accused of being witches were actually professional wise women, healers and midwives, how many were 'ordinary women' and how many were practicing witches, and what powers and skills they may have truly had. I am sure that many a woman healer and herbalist, and anyone who held pagan beliefs or folk practices was pulled into some of the fictional imagery that saw them transformed into a witch or sorceress. There is power, skill and meaning here in these histories, traditions held on to that are worth protecting and celebrating, especially, because so many suffered on the journey, and so many stories have already been carelessly lost and forgotten.

THE WITCH'S KITCHEN

The craft of the real witch is not nearly as dramatic as their fictional kin, no flying through the air, no sparks from the cauldron (well, maybe just a few!). The day-to-day practices of real witches are healing, cooking, listening, connecting, knowing – this is the 'ordinary' magic that moves us through our days. Much of this happens in kitchens. In the simplest of positive connections, the kitchen is where many witches work their magic.[*]

The kitchen has always been part of the story of the witch. And whilst the idea of calling someone or something a Kitchen Witch is relatively modern, the magic and the archetype of the witch's kitchen is ancient. This archetype of the wise woman cooking up magic in her cauldron, creating recipes of the esoteric at her hearth is timeless. Names and ways of telling the story may change, but the magic of the Kitchen Witch, I think, has always been there.

The witch has tightly wound links with rural customs and the practices of the poor. It may have been that a witch could not often afford the luxury of butter

---

[*] Not everyone calls this magic, you might think of it as connection to an energy, intuition, flow, spirit, universe: I will leave this up to you to consider.

(though many superstitions say she steals it), hence animal fat and oils might be present in the witch's kitchen, as well as the least favourable parts of animals: tripe, offal, maybe even skin and eyes – nothing would be wasted. Often the recipes of a societies' poorest members are about making the most of 'leftover' parts of animals, so sometimes there really were bones floating in witches' cauldrons (and still are today, for a good stock). But this is also testament to the witches' tenacity and their extraordinary work through time: they may have worked in darkness, the cold and damp and in poverty – still, they brought magic. The real power of the witch in the kitchen is to see and know the healing abilities of the humble: bringing together scattered, foraged or meagre ingredients together into a warming meal that will nourish, heal and comfort. That's real magic.

The witch's story, including superstitions about her, is tied in with how and what ordinary folks had to do to survive. She is associated with foods that she had the skills to gather for free from the hedgerows such as nuts, berries and mushrooms, as well as with medicinal and aromatic herbs sought in wild fields or grown in the garden, which were used for herbal teas and infusions. Together, these formed a major part of the kitchen pharmacy of the time and the only medicines accessible to most people.

The chief strength of poor witches lies in the gathering and boiling of herbs. The most esteemed herbs for their purposes are the Betony-root, Henbane, Mandrake, Deadly Nightshade, Origanum, Antirrhinum, female Phlox, Arum, Red and White Celandine, Millefoil, Horned Poppy, Fern, Adder's-tongue, and ground Ivy. Root of Hemlock, "digged in the dark," slips of Yew, "slivered in the moon's eclipse," Cypress, Wild Fig, Larch, Broom, and Thorn are also associated with Witches and their necromancy. The divining Gall-apple of the Oak, the mystic Mistletoe, the Savin, the Moonwort, the Vervain, and the St. John's Wort are considered magical, and therefore form part of the Witches' pharmacopœia – to be produced as occasion may require, and their juices infused in the hell-broths, philtres, potions, and baleful draughts prepared for their enemies.

Richard Folkard, *Plant Lore, Legends, and Lyrics* (1884)

Part of the rural cook, healer, and Kitchen Witch's apothecary could well have included plants like poppy, mandrake, hemlock and belladonna: powerful ingredients all capable of causing hallucinations, visions and capable of poisoning in the wrong hands. Many such formidable herbs and plants would come to be permanently connected to the witch, and approached, like her, with some trepidation.

THE FIRST KITCHEN WITCHES

A "Kitchen Witch" uses magick (thaumaturgy) to help handle the details of daily life – for example, to keep a household running smoothly. The ritual tools of this practice are the tools of everyday life: a paring knife for an athame, a carved potato for a healing poppet. "Rituals" are simple, almost casual, in appearance.

Amber K, *True Magick: a beginner's guide* **(1990)**

We find the Kitchen Witch (by varied names) from the classical stories of goddesses round cauldrons in ancient Rome and Greece, to paintings that depict Faust and Macbeth, moving into popular culture, in poem, craft and cookbooks: Vianne Rocher in *Chocolat* and Tita in *Like Water for Chocolate,* whose emotions are woven through their cooking, as well as the pancakes and midnight margaritas of the Owens sisters in *Practical Magic* (some of the best food references come from the film rather than the book, but both are delightful!).

As I tried to trace the history of the Kitchen Witch, I fell into many a rabbit hole of research, trawling through old newspapers of the 1850's advertising a range of *Kitchen Witch* ovens, to names for cafés and catering companies, articles on fictional Kitchen Witches and pictures of straw Kitchen Witches hung in colonial kitchens in America.

We don't know precisely when the term Kitchen Witch first became known and used when referring to a person, but we see the term edging into common usage in the 1500s to refer to a type of poppet or homemade protective doll. Often referenced is a line of text from the will of John Croginton from Newton Shropshire in England, dated 1599, in which he divides his belongings amongst his wife and children:

> *I give and bequeath to my sonne John and hys heyres forever to be heirloomes the things hereafter nexte of first mentyoned, that ys to saye, one witche in the kytchyn, one weeting fatte, one kneadynge knive[...]except the cubbard in the halle the witche in the kytchyn which I gyve and bequeathe to Roger my sonne.*[3]

This could be referring to a Kitchen Witch poppet, but we really don't know. To me, this begs the question of how and why this man valued and remembers the "witche" particularly and why he wanted his son to have it. Did he have two, hence offering one up to both John and Roger? At this time, the kitchen would have still been a woman's realm, so I wonder if it was a keepsake of his mother or a female relative.

Kitchen Witch Poppets

A Kitchen Witch poppet or doll, sometimes called a Cottage Witch, is placed in kitchens as a good luck charm. The Kitchen Witch was thought to prevent kitchen mishaps, countering perhaps the mischief of spirits who curdled milk, would not allow bread to rise, burned food, and made pots boil over. She was also kept to inspire creativity in the cook.

More than one country claims to be the home of the Kitchen Witch poppet, including Germany, Norway and Sweden. Made to resemble a stereotypical hag or crone, she may be clad in the black robes and hat of a Halloween witch, but can also be seen in a bright apron and head scarf. She often rides a broom, a wooden spoon, a whisk or other kitchen implement.

The Kitchen Witch may hold cutesy and quaint associations for those who know her only from her kitchen dolly decoration incarnation, all frilly aprons, lavender bundles and cinnamon cookies. But in her story lies the powerful priestesses of bread and beer, the cruelly maligned alewives and herbwives, and rituals to appease fierce goddesses. Marketing for Kitchen Witch poppets from the 1960s and 70s suggests that the tradition is centuries old, and we know both that charms have been hung in kitchens for millennia, and that poppets are ancient magic.

In folk magic and witchcraft, poppets are dolls made to represent people, animals, spirits or deities. One may use them to cast spells, seek favour, and ward off bad luck.[*] This is craft based on sympathetic or image magic, a practice dating back to prehistoric times.

Examples of poppets around the world include the *kolossoi* from ancient Greece to Haitian *vodou* dolls. In the British Isles, they are still occasionally found lodged in chimneys or in the walls of homes. The Museum of Witchcraft and Magic in Cornwall has an excellent collection of such poppets, and it is one of their most popular displays. The surviving poppets found are made of such things as wax, clay, grain stalks or cloth.

---

[*] To ward off bad luck, misfortune or evil spirits is also known as apotropaic magic – which can take such forms as poppets, charms, spells and rituals, and dressing up for Halloween to scare off wandering spirits...

In a book called *The Story of My Life* by Ellen Terry (1908), she speaks of her adventures in acting, and she mentions one of the players for *Faust* switching roles to play "the Kitchen Witch." Although she doesn't go into any more detail, we know in the story of *Faust*, a classic German legend of a man who does a deal with the Devil and in the Goethe version, visits the kitchen of a witch to obtain a potion of youth. This scene of Faust in the witch's kitchen is the subject of many classical artworks. In fact, you'll find many paintings depicting and/or named 'The Witch's Kitchen,' artists it seems, were just as fascinated as the rest of us as to what went on in the steam and smoke of this place of magic.

So, we have evidence that Kitchen Witch was a term that has been applied to people, as well as poppets for well over a century (and for the phrase to pop up in writing means it's most likely a term that is already well-known.)

When I posed the question on various social media platforms, some people mentioned their grandmothers calling themselves Kitchen Witches in the 1960s and 1970s. And by the 1990's, it was appearing in books on Wicca, magic and as subject for magical cookbooks like Patricia Telesco's *A Kitchen Witch's Cookbook* (1994). The term was joyfully claimed both by practitioners of witchcraft and home cooks. From then the Kitchen Witch really took flight as a pathway of magical practice, and was claimed as positive. The magical work done in the kitchen and the named poppets came together to represent a witch who uses or focuses on traditional practices of the home.

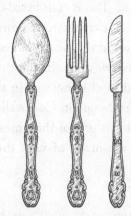

WOMEN OF THE CAULDRON

Double, double toil and trouble; Fire burn, and cauldron bubble.
William Shakespeare, *Macbeth* (1606)

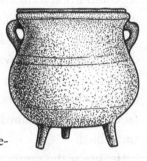

Cooking pots, cauldrons and the hearth fire were, for millennia, the centre of a household. Women were, and often still are, bearers of family knowledge and traditions, family customs, tribal lore which centred around cauldron and fire, and many deities of the homestead are depicted as female, watching over the most precious elements of home and family.

In Karl Pearson's essay "Woman as Witch" (1897), he calls the folklore and superstitions of the spinning wheel, cauldron and broom and their connected deities and feasts "fossils of the *mother-age*." As we shall see, these "fossils" were often either adopted by the Church, or cast into dark corners and called witchcraft.

The cauldron has, over time, gathered a rich wealth of folklore associated with it. All sorts of magics were thought to come from the cooking pot – from Siris, Babylonian goddess of fate and sky mother who stirs her cauldron made of lapis lazuli, to Welsh goddess Branwen, whose cauldron of regeneration could hold a dead man and resurrect him by morning, to the Greek oracles of Delphi and Dodona that sat in three-legged cauldrons amongst steam and smoke that allowed them to travel to other realms of consciousness.

The cauldron represents many things in folklore, as a symbol of the mother goddess, the womb, nourishment, heat, regeneration, time, fate, transformation, and creation. The following are just some of the many stories of the goddesses and women of the cauldron, who stand around it, and sometimes in it!

CELTIC CAULDRONS:
KERRIDWEN AND BRIGID

In Celtic lore, cauldrons can contain an unending supply of knowledge or food. In the stories of Welsh goddess Kerridwen, she is the Keeper of the Cauldron as a place of divine healing and transformation, in which knowledge and inspiration are brewed. Those who taste of this brew will at once understand the secrets of creation and of all time.

Because of her great knowledge and insight, Kerridwen is almost always depicted as a crone, a wise woman of healing, and rightly so, as time and age are our greatest tools in gathering wisdom, experience and inspiration. Kerridwen continually stirs the spirals of life within the cauldron, where inspiration and divine knowledge swirl alongside the eternal cycle of birth, death and rebirth.

The fire at the centre of the home provided physical and social warmth as the family gathered around it. The cauldrons not owned by goddesses, would sit at the household fire: a place sacred to the Irish goddess Brigid. She, the "bright one," is often depicted as a fire herself or with a divine flame rising from her head and watches over all things hearth and kitchen related.

Brigid's father was Dagda, a revered leader of the Tuatha Dé Danann.* Associated with agriculture, strength and knowledge, he carried a huge magic cauldron that was bottomless, representing abundance and Dagda's own penchant for food. I think part of the role of host passed through from father to daughter. To be with Dagda is to never go hungry, and to be with Brigid is to always be warmed. (She also brought the beer – I'll come back to that shortly!)

The close links between hearth and healing are present in the image of Brigid. I think you can see here how ancient Celts took everything that fire and hearth meant to them and created these glorious deities to embody that light, warmth and comfort the hearth fire provided. The goddesses' skills connect to what happened around hearth fires. At the hearth, the women of the house practiced magic, cooking, storytelling and healing, as well as the passing on of knowledge. It was around the hearth that wisdom was passed from one generation to the next and stories were shared, something we will return to later in this chapter.

---

* The supernatural predecessors of the Irish people in Irish mythology.

ANCIENT GREEK CAULDRONS:
HECATE, MEDEA AND CIRCE

A sorceress, witch, priestess of Hecate (goddess of magic and witches) and guardian of the Cauldron of Rejuvenation, images of Medea and her cauldron feature in ancient Greek pottery dating back to 600 BCE, and representations of Hecate date back a further century.

Medea, whose name means "to devise," used magical formulae to achieve control over life and death, to rejuvenate and resurrect. In stories of Medea, we see the boiling of the limbs in a cauldron filled with all manner of herbs, which no doubt had an effect on later depictions of women at cauldrons. According to myth, Medea first demonstrated her skills by transforming herself from an old woman into a beautiful young one. Jason, of the Argonauts, sought her out to restore the youth of his aged father. She prepared a potion of henbane to give to Jason to make him impervious to pain whilst searching for the Golden Fleece, but uses belladonna when she attempts to poison and kill Theseus.

Medea's aunt, Circe, is another great sorceress in Greek mythology who would have stood at the edge of cauldrons. Daughter of the sun god Helios (and in some tales Hecate herself), Circe was renowned for her knowledge of potions and herbs and in *The Odyssey*, transforms Odysseus' companions into animals by feeding them a magic potion mixed into a drink made of honey and wine.

Roman lyric poet Horace (65-8 BCE) draws on the Greek tradition of witchcraft – Medea's potions, Circe's spells, and Hecate's place in the Underworld – when he writes about Canidia in several poems as both making love potions and putting bodies into cauldrons. She resembles all of them, but not their connections to divinity. Canidia is not a goddess, but rather a real woman with magical powers: what we would call a witch.

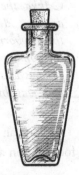

HOUSEHOLD GODS AND SPIRITS

For centuries, Kitchen Witches have called upon native deities or sought favour from household spirits within the home itself for blessing, assistance and protection. The Kitchen Witch may visit the gods of the old Roman temples, or tell tales of Germanic deities whose stories had travelled with the Saxons. She may use spirits of the land around her home – trees and elements or local stories passed down through generations. She may have charms, herbs or sigils around her home or advise others how to use them.

The presence of many deities and spirits within the home and land, which could be represented in statues, symbols and directly petitioned is at odds with Christian belief of the One True God of Christianity, judging from on high. This is, no doubt, one reason why the witch and her many deities were seen as a threat to patriarchal religions, a threat that needed to be violently destroyed.

There are many traditional gods and goddesses of food, home and harvest around the world. *In Sacred Home: Creating Shelter for Your Soul* (2004), Laurine Morrison Meyer shares just some of those popular in Europe:

In Lithuania, Aspelenie ruled the corner of the house behind the door, and Gabija, goddess of the hearth was honored by throwing salt into the flames. Malergabiae was a Fire goddess of the Lithuanian house, and the first loaf of bread was offered to her. Women used their fingers to indent the dough as a sign that the loaf was dedicated to her. Baba Yaga was a Slavic kitchen witch who lived in the last sheaf of grain, known to bring good fortune to the families she protected. A Celtic goddess of the horse and dog, Epona, was depicted with the cornucopia and the key which signified abundance and nurture. Haltia was the Baltic Finnish spirit who lived in the roof beams, kept an eye on the house, and stood guard over the family's wealth. Madder Akka, the Swedish goddess of birth and women's fertility, one of her aspects as Uks Akka, the Old Lady of the Door, was present at births to receive the newborn baby. She lived beneath the threshold, blessing all those who left the home, much like the newborn leaving the womb. In Siberia, the hearth goddess was Poza-Mama, who kept the family warm. The first morsel of food was thrown into the fire in an offering to her.

As you can see there was a veritable pantheon of domestic deities! I will be focusing on a few of the goddesses and house spirits from the European tradition – ancient Greek and Roman, Celtic and Anglo-Saxon, as we nurture and nourish the feminine on this journey. There are many ideas for further reading at the back of the book if you would like to explore further.

GREEK DEITIES: HESTIA AND DEMETER

Hestia is goddess of fire, the domestic hearth and the guardian spirit of home life. In ancient Greece, the hearth was regarded as the most important and most sacred place in the home: the fire was the source of heat, protection and nourishment, the centre of every house. Round this domestic hearth, family members would gather, prayers might be said, and sacrifices offered. Hestia's name means hearth, fire, and altar; sacred hearth fires were constantly tended within her temples, and offerings of sweet wine and food made in her name. As patroness of the hearth fire, Hestia watched over the daily activities of baking bread, preparing meals and, in turn, the health of the family.

She reminds us of the centrality of the kitchen witchery of cooking, cleaning and making a house a home that goes on quietly in the background of busy, noisy lives. To tend your hearth is not always a big and adventurous undertaking – but it is beautiful and vital magic.

Hestia's sister is Demeter. She, too, holds connections to the home.

Demeter is the goddess of the harvested grain contained within much of the food cooked within the home. As grains created bread and cereal, they were symbols of both survival and bounty. In ancient Rome she was called Ceres. Ceres, like Demeter, was the goddess of agriculture. Romans had an expression, "fit for Ceres," which meant something very fine, magnificent enough for the goddess.

Demeter passed the art of growing and using corn onto mortals and is often portrayed in artworks as holding corn or bedecked with a corn crown, flowers and fruit, blessing the earth with fertile soils and good harvests. The favour of Demeter was believed to bring rich harvests and fruitful crops, whereas her displeasure caused blight, drought, and famine.

Fertility was an uncertainty. It was never guaranteed that a harvest would turn out well, and the same goes for conception and childbirth, so the goddesses' blessings would be sought for hope and comfort. Many of the Greek gods had, at one point or another, their own festivals, and for Demeter it was Thesmophoria, a fertility festival attended only by women and lasting several days, including fasting, feasting and offerings to the goddess. Demeter's daughter Persephone was also closely connected with the Thesmophoria, with rituals that commemorated marriage, fertility, family and the abduction and return of Persephone. (The descent and rise of Persephone and her mother Demeter were also at the centre of a collection of rituals known as the Eleusinian Mysteries.)

Dinner with Hecate

Hecate (also known as Hekate) is a witch-goddess associated with crossroads and the Underworld, gateways, night-time, magic and witchcraft. With a great knowledge of herbs and poisonous plants, she was one of several deities worshipped in ancient Greece as a protector of the Oikos (household), alongside Hestia, and other gods such as Hermes, Zeus, and Apollo.

Each Greek luni-solar month ended with three days of special ritual and celebrations allowing families to step into a new month with a sense of hope. The new moon was the last day of the lunar month, and the time for cleansing the household with incense carried through rooms, and the clearing away of the fire ashes, leftovers, offerings or food fallen on the floor (not to be eaten, as it belongs to Hecate at this point). One would also atone for any bad deeds that may have offended Hecate (which may include animal sacrifice), causing her to withhold her favour, and the offering of Hecate's *Deipnon*.

In ancient Greece *deipnon* was the evening meal. Hecate's *Deipnon* was a sacred meal offered to the goddess at new moon. Offerings were intended to appease not only this goddess and seek her blessing for prosperous daily life, but as goddess of the Underworld, this was also an appeasing of any restless spirits and beings in her company, that may seek to cross boundaries from the Underworld. On the night of the new moon, a ritual would take place and a meal would be set outside. Food offerings might include cake or bread, fish, eggs and honey. In households this would be laid out in a small shrine to Hecate by the front door, as the street in front of the house and the doorway create a crossroads, known to be a place Hecate dwelled.

The next nightfall was celebrated as the *Noumenia*, the first day on the new lunar month, when the first sliver of moon may be visible. It was held in honour of moon goddess Selene, Hestia and the other household gods. This ritual period would end with a chance to honour the *agathos daimon* (good/noble spirit) as well as one's own personal spirit. Often a libation would be set at the family altar and prayer offered to seek continued blessings for one's self and family.

Due to roaming spirits, Greeks might stay within their homes during the night hours of the dark moon. There are some elements of real fear and importance to these rituals and ceremonies, based around belief: it was serious stuff to protect your family from furious gods, evil spirits and vengeful ghosts.

ROMAN DEITIES:
VESTA, FORNAX AND THE LARES

Vesta was Hestia's counterpart in ancient Rome, and her priestesses, the Vestal Virgins, were charged with keeping the sacred fire burning in her temples. Often home hearths would be ceremoniously relit from this central sacred fire (a practice that can also be seen in Celtic traditions for fire festivals like Beltane and Samhain). Vesta's flame and temples were regarded as fundamental to the security and dominance of the Empire. For Vestalia, her festival, priestesses gathered grain and baked cakes made from fine salted flour. This was also sprinkled on the heads of animals to be sacrificed, on altars and in sacred fires.

Related to bread and baking we have the divine personification of the oven: the goddess Fornax, the 'Oven Mother.' Her festival, the Fornacalia, was celebrated in February. Bread and cakes featured heavily in many Roman religious rites, and when the weather was cold and dark, warm bread fresh out of the oven must have felt like a real blessing. During the festival, ovens were draped in garlands, spelt and grains were toasted and offered to Fornax, in order that she bless the ovens for the coming year. Her priestesses were called the "Ladies of Bread."

Rome, like many cultures at that time, was polytheistic: a culture that worshipped many, many gods and goddesses. The Romans managed to find a god for everything relating to food. So, I could mention Edesia here, to squeeze in more goddesses! She is the divine spirit of feasting, which was considered such a magical and important act by the Romans to be deserving of its own goddess! She blesses banquets, according to the sacrifices made by the host, and is accompanied by her sister Bibesia, the goddess of drink. Her name comes from the Latin *bibi*, "to drink, toast, or visit," the root of our modern English word imbibe "to drink in." She personified the divine spirit of the drink or wine served at the table and was perhaps believed to make sure both that the wine was of good quality and that it flowed freely. Grand offerings were thought to assure the presence and blessing of these two goddesses.

The Lares were the watchmen, guardian and benevolent ancestor spirits of homes and hearths in ancient Rome, thought to directly affect a family's home and daily life. They dwelled, among other places, under the hearth in their family's household and were sometimes depicted in snake or lizard form (animals that would have regularly popped up around homes in the Mediterranean). Images of the Lares in human and animal form, and Vesta can be seen in remains of shrines to the Lares (also called lararium) in the ruined Ancient Roman cities of Pompeii and Herculaneum.

The Lares required acknowledgement and honouring to ensure one's family prospered. There might be a shrine in the home, and how well the people of the house treated their spirits was mirrored in the household's fortunes. Homes in which rituals and spirits were kept with devotion would thrive. Daily prayers would be given, alongside offerings such as milk, honey and wine, with more elaborate rituals on special days. Offerings for the Lares might also be placed at boundary points like doorways, windows and at the hearth chimney where the Lares may guard, as spirits and energy; good and bad may appear in these places of the in-between.

Panes or Penates were the spirits specifically of the pantry and the kitchen, making sure the household was never in want of food and that the food within was protected. Icons were set on the table during meals, thanks given to them before eating, and a portion of the meal set aside in their honour or burned in the hearth fire as a ritual offering.

House Spirits

Household deities or spirits like the Lares may protect a home or look after the household, or they may have more mischievous or opportunist intentions. It is a belief in paganism, as well as in folklore across many parts of the world, that ancestors as well as domestic goddesses reside in groups in homes, watching over the family. So, families may well feel a more personal connection to household spirits, as ancestors of the family or land, and they would be honoured, not in temples but within the home.

Some examples of these spirits in European cultures include:

☾ Fairies – also known as fae, faery, fair folk and fae folk (throughout the British Isles)

☾ The *coblynau* – mine fairies and *bwbachod* – household fairies (Welsh)

☾ Bogeys, *bwg*, goblins (Welsh)

☾ Elves (English)

☾ *Huldufólk* – Hidden Folk (Icelandic)

☾ Brownies (Scottish and English)

☾ Leprechauns and clúrichauns (Irish)

☾ Bogles (Scottish)

☾ Piskies (Cornish)

☾ *Kobolds* (Germany)

☾ Hobgoblins and pixies (England)

☾ *Nisse* (Norwegian and Danish)

☾ *Tomte* (Swedish)

☾ *Tonttu* (Finnish)

Because of their place within the home, house spirits were connected to the day-to-day goings-on and chores. House spirits are often considered to clean, tidy and protect the home in exchange for milk, bread or cake. They are also part of deeply woven together ideas of witches and fairies and night-flying spirits. So we will meet many fairy folk through the book, and vestiges of their presence persisting in small ways, into the modern day.

A bowl of milk placed for the brownie is not so different to an offering of wine poured out before the household gods of the Romans. Fairy lore contains certain elements of mythology and of older religious beliefs. I believe fairies reflect remnants of pagan beliefs of animism – that all objects, places, and creatures possess a distinct energy or spirit. Animism perceives all things – plants, rocks, rivers, homes, words and food – as alive in some way, possessing a certain magic, you might say.

Hobgoblin and Bogles

"Hob" is a generic term given to a goblin, bogle or brownie. A hob is also a shelf by a fireplace for heating pans, which means that a hobgoblin may be referring to a household goblin or spirit that resides in this particular location in the kitchen. Hobgoblins may help with cleaning and housework in return for food, however, if offended, they could become disruptive and mischievous. There is a story of a bogle who would hide in potato fields of Scotland – the Tatty Bogle might attack unwary humans or cause blight to the crop.

Kobold

The *kobolds* of German folklore hold many similarities with the hobgoblin – they may help with chores but are just as likely to be mischievous and hide household tools. Like similar incarnations in other countries, he becomes outraged if he is not properly fed. *Kobolds* dwell in dark and solitary places, basement and storerooms and further afield in mines and tunnels.

Bienal is a *kobold* of the beer cellar, like the leprechauns and clurichauns in Ireland – there often seems to be a spirit specifically for booze (even whisky has its own angels – we'll meet them later). The *bienal* is appeased by a daily jug of beer, and in return might assist in cleaning tables and washing up. Finally, for our stop in Germany, numerous demons are recognized as dwelling in trees and amongst the crops of wheat and vegetables. So, amongst the *Feldgeister* "field spirits," you will find: the *Roggenhund* – rye dog, the *Kornkatze* – corn cat, and *Kartoffelwolf* – potato wolf.

Piskies

Fairy folk local to Cornwall, piskies are often sighted at places of ancient worship, such as stone circles and barrows. There are many tales attached to who the piskies are: the souls of pagans who could not ascend to heaven, ancestor spirits, relics of pagan gods or nature spirits… even moths, who some believe to be departed souls, are still in some areas, called piskies.

They can also be mischievous, and if you get lost, the Cornish might say you were "piskie-led," although people are often lead astray in order to join in with dancing and games before being returned to their path, so it's not all bad!

The piskies of the Cornish Moors are also called nightriders for their hobby of knotting tiny stirrups into the manes of moorland horses and galloping across the moors. Horses ridden by witches in similar stories are called "hag-ridden."

Piskies might also blow out candles or stop milk from being churned to butter or sneak through keyholes to eat sweet food. But there are also plenty of stories of very kind acts of the piskies. One tale tells of the piskies who sent to the Earl of Cornwall's wife – who longed for a baby – a pie, within which lay, on a bed of sweet herbs and wildflowers, a smiling infant.

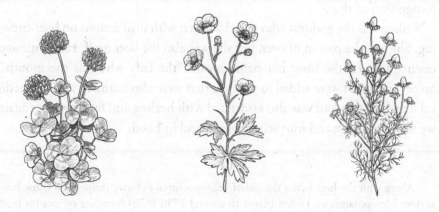

FROM BEER GODDESSES TO ALEWIVES

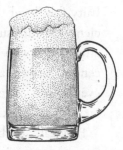

Throughout history, beer was used for religious ritual, medicine, nourishment and as a day-to-day beverage.

When we journey through the story of beer, there are more goddesses, but also many real women standing at their cauldrons. The legacy of woman as brewer persisted from ancient times well into the Middle Ages across many different cultures.

THE FIRST BREWERS

Ancient Sumerian settlements, located in Mesopotamia, are credited with the invention of farming, written language…and beer. In fact, the oldest known beer recipe in the world sits on a clay tablet in cuneiform writing. It is called, in translation, "A Hymn to Ninkasi" and is a glimpse into beer's ancient history, a beautiful ode etched into clay (1800 BCE).[*]

Ancient Sumeria was a patriarchal society, and women held significantly fewer rights than men. And yet we know it was women, most likely priestesses (who were thought to have sacred connections to the deities) who made this beer. They made it both for, and with the help of, the goddess Ninkasi. In brewing beer, these ancient women had an opportunity to both make a living and hold a position of respect: "The Hymn to Ninkasi" represents a recognition of that.

Ninkasi was the goddess who gifted women with instructions on beer-brewing. She was the patron of beer, but she was also the beer itself. Her spirit and essence infused the beer: her name means "the lady who fills the mouth." Spices and herbs were added to the beer that were also found in ancient medical remedies. Ninkasi was also associated with healing and fertility, once again we see nourishing and nurturing going hand in hand.

---

[*] Along with the beer hymn the oldest known written culinary recipes also come from ancient Mesopotamia on tablets (dated to around 1750 BCE) featuring recipes for lamb stew and soup with leek and garlic, they are kept in the archives of Yale University.

Sumerian women brewed beer in, and as, ceremony. In the following translation of the "Hymn to Ninkasi," woven between the hypnotic words are detailed instructions for brewing beer, a sacred, feminine, life-sustaining craft. You get a sense of the song, movements and rhythm that would have been part of making this drink for their goddess. Most lines are repeated twice, in a call and response type format.

Hymn to Ninkasi[†]

Borne of the flowing water,
Tenderly cared for by the Ninhursag,[‡]
Borne of the flowing water,
Tenderly cared for by the Ninhursag,
Having founded your town by the sacred lake,
[...]
You are the one who soaks the malt in a jar,
The waves rise, the waves fall.
Ninkasi, you are the one who soaks the malt in a jar,
The waves rise, the waves fall.
You are the one who spreads the cooked mash on large reed mats,
Coolness overcomes,
Ninkasi, you are the one who spreads the cooked mash on large reed mats,
Coolness overcomes,
You are the one who holds with both hands the great sweet wort,
Brewing it with honey and wine
You the sweet wort to the vessel
Ninkasi, You the sweet wort to the vessel
The filtering barrel, which makes a pleasant sound,
You place well on top of a great barrel.
[...]
Ninkasi, you are the one who pours out the filtered beer from the barrel,
Like the flow of Tigris and Euphrates.

---

† This translation is drawn from several academic versions.
‡ An earth goddess figure and "Lady of the Mountain."

In ancient Egypt, beermaking was also woman's work, it followed a method similar to Sumerian beer, often using dough as a base for both beer and bread, and was undertaken by the priestesses of the goddess Tjenenet, who watched over beer brewing (and the lives of women). Her name may have derived from the word *tenemu* meaning beer. Another goddess, Hathor, was considered to have invented brewing processes. She and her temple at Dendera were connected to the experience of drunkenness and intoxication. Various carvings and hieroglyphics have been found depicting women both brewing and drinking the beverage. Other myths also draw in Osiris, Isis and Nephthys as connected to beer as well: truly it was considered a very blessed gift.

From beer and barley wine recorded through Mesopotamia and Egypt, the brewing process, and stories of goddesses that watched over it, spread through Africa and beyond. Ancient Greeks and Romans enjoyed wine and *cervisia* (beer). All through Europe, as people travelled, so did fermented drinks. Just like in Mesopotamia, Sumer and Egypt, the brewer's craft was the provenance of women who brewed beer in the home to supplement the daily meals (and ensure something safe to drink). Across cultures, brewing was a medium for magic, guarded and blessed by both women and gods.

Aegir, the Norse god of the sea, is credited with brewing the best beer in the Nine Realms and for hosting festivities for the other gods, where all were plied with plentiful amounts of beer. However, there is a feminine presence here too, as he was assisted by nine daughters, known as the wave or billow maidens, who brewed the ale in a giant cauldron.

Women used their knowledge of herbs and plants in their brewing. In Finland, women created recipes containing hops, juniper twigs, along with barley and rye grains. Archaeologists have uncovered graves of pre-Viking Nordic people that show some of the herbs in use. In the Danish peat bog grave of the "Egtved Girl," a bucket buried at her feet, made of birch, showed that the drink was made from a mixture of wheat as a base and included cranberries, honey, and lingonberries, as well as herbs, including bog myrtle.

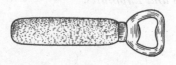

The Beer Witch

In the Finnish epic *Kalevala* (1835), it's beer witches and magical maidens all round – the Mistress of the North, witch Louhi, needs beer for the great wedding of her daughter, the Maiden of the Rainbow, so she seeks the help of Osmotar, the Finnish goddess of beer who creates a magical ale with "heart-easing" honey that sparkles and overflows from cauldrons, with the help of "mystic maidens" Kalevatar and Kapo, and a bee who takes a trip into honey-fields of magic.

> *In the honey-fields of magic;*
> *By her side were honeyed grasses,*
> *By her lips were fragrant flowers,*
> *Silver stalks with golden petals;*
> *Dipped its winglets in the honey,*
> *Dipped its fingers in the juices*
> *Of the sweetest of the flowers,*
> *Brought the honey back to Kapo,*
> *To the mystic maiden's fingers.*
> *Osmotar, the beer-preparer,*
> *Placed the honey in the liquor;*
> *Kapo mixed the beer and honey,*
> *And the wedding-beer fermented;*
> *Rose the live beer upward, upward,*
> *From the bottom of the vessels,*
> *Upward in the tubs of birch-wood,*
> *Foaming higher, higher, higher,*
> *Till it touched the oaken handles,*
> *Overflowing all the caldrons;*
> *To the ground it foamed and sparkled,*
> *Sank away in sand and gravel.*[*]

---

[*] English translation: *Kalevala: The Epic poem of Finland*, John Martin Crawford (1888). The story of Kalevala is much more complex than just this small part, and is full of delights, but it's too long for me to include the full text here. Read the whole thing at sentiayoga.com/kitchenwitch

The use of hops in beer as a preservative is most often credited to St. Hildegard von Bingen (1098–1179), a fascinating wise woman who was, among other things: a German Benedictine abbess, writer, philosopher, mystic and musician (and was officially made a saint in the twenty-first century). Monasteries in Europe took on the production of alcoholic beverages around the eleventh century, along with growing herbal gardens and writing manuscripts from old texts. Hildegard brought all these skills together in her work, writing books on health and healing with plants and food. But along with her support of hops, she did also say that this information wouldn't be useful to men, and that they should avoid beer altogether as it "makes the soul of man sad."

St. Brigid's Brew

Brigid is another goddess connected to beer. In her form as Christian saint, she is patron saint of beer and brewing. In her more primal Celtic goddess form she offers the gift of ale to humankind, ale of such quality that one who drank it may become immortal – so strong stuff! – however, Brigid may withhold beer from the greedy and selfish, which seems fair to me.

There is a story that she could turn water into beer. Nowadays, we just call that process brewing, but it takes a little longer than Brigid's miracle beer, and she could not only turn water into beer for the poor, but beer back into the water for the uncharitable. There are tales that Brigid can, and does, transform everything from well water to her own bathwater into beer. In a classic tale of making much nourishment from very little, she once made beer enough for seventeen churches' celebrations from meagre household stores.

One of my favourite stories of Brigid and booze is that she was accidentally ordained as a bishop because, apparently, the church official was drunk. This made her the first woman bishop in history. You can see in this account from the early ninth century *Bethu Brigte*, a biography of Brigid:

The bishop being intoxicated with the grace of God there did not recognise what he was reciting from his book, for he consecrated Brigit with the orders of a Bishop. This virgin alone in Ireland, said Mel, will hold the Episco-

pal ordination. While she was being consecrated a fiery column ascended from her head.

Afterwards, Bishop Mel was asked why he had read the incorrect prayers making Brigid a bishop. He replied that the Holy Spirit had taken the matter out of his hands: the jury is still out on the nature of this "spirit"!

ALEWIVES

The stories of the beer goddess offer us a glimpse of just how essential a role beer and ale have played over many thousands of years of feasting, ritual and daily life – and how women have always played a central role in its production. The word "alewife" appeared in use in England from the end of the 1300s in various medieval texts to describe women who brewed and sold ale. Brewing was something done at home for the household, but especially for widows and spinsters brewing a little extra for sale was a good way to earn some income. And many were familiar with herbs and flavourings that might make the ale taste better, as well as containing healing properties. Apparently, ale was particularly useful after The Black Death (around 1346–1352, which wiped out between one-third to one-half of Europe's population). As it was boiled, ale was more likely safer to drink than water in some areas, it provided some nutrition and hydration.

Professional alewives would have broomsticks in their kitchen to keep things clean, cats often scurried around their bubbling cauldrons killing mice that liked to feast on the grains used for brewing or warming themselves by cauldrons of cooling wort. The frothing yeast from the pot might be skimmed and added to flour, for the baking of bread that day. If this image is sounding familiar, it's because this is all iconography that we now associate with witches. While there's no definitive historical proof that modern depictions of witches were modelled after 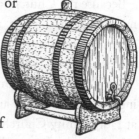 alewives, there are some uncanny similarities between alewives and anti-witch propaganda. And as brewing gradually moved from a cottage industry into a money-making one, this connection to witchcraft proved useful for men to remove women and their roles with demonisation and character assassination. Other skills such as lay healers suffered a similar fate, and women were stripped of their ability to claim a profession or have their skills recognised. Medicinal knowledge was considered impossible for a woman to possess, therefore her skills must have been begotten by the Devil.

As the idea that women brewers were innately corrupt spread, they were increasingly regulated and removed from the trade. Brewing guilds were set up in cities and excluded women, as they were considered unfit to brew or sell ale and beer, or worse, that they might use their feminine charms to lure men into drunkenness or poison them. Throughout Europe, the founding of these guilds often forced women in towns and cities out of the brewing industry. However, it was still possible for women in rural villages to continue their craft, albeit more surreptitiously.

Your Mother Serves Pints in Hell

The medieval Church was not a fan of the alewife either. They saw these early female entrepreneurs as temptresses who used their wiles to get men drunk and spend money. The Church saw alehouses as playgrounds for the Devil and encouragers of the cardinal sins of gluttony and lust. The demonisation of women as immoral witches and the forced association of paganism with Devil worship meant that women became the apex of the blame for overindulgence in alcohol. And many an over-indulger may have blamed their inappropriate behaviour on the women brewers, accusing them of being under a spell.

Because the Church loves a good, angry story about hell, they began commissioning art known as doom paintings. These were murals on walls and ceilings depicting poor disobedient souls condemned to various realms of hell. And who should feature heavily in these images? The alewife, of course.

You'll find doom paintings and carvings around England of alewives hanging out with demons and in various hellscapes at St. Laurence's in Ludlow, at Holy Trinity Church in Coventry and St. Thomas's, Salisbury. An alewife rides piggy-back on a demon as they cart a human off to hell on the ceiling of Norwich Cathedral. I feel this is a good body of proof that alewives were disliked by the Church in general. They seem to be depicted in hell with some regularity, and generally in a similar manner: naked and holding a tankard of ale – an extreme vision of all women's potential failings, providing justification for barring women from both brewing and taverns altogether. Poems and songs insulting alewives included physical insults such as a hooked nose, warts on her face, long spindly fingers and crooked back as well as suggesting they cheat, lie, steal and seduce. Slowly but surely, Europeans came to see alewives not as legitimate business owners doing a service for their community, but as immoral women in league with the Devil himself.

According to Essex witch trial records, accused witches were quite often blamed for spoiling beer, or using powers to "bewitch" beer, which could, among other things, mean it was watered down. The connection between women brewers and untrustworthy magics stuck, accusing alewives of witchcraft became a weapon, and this ancient tradition was broken.

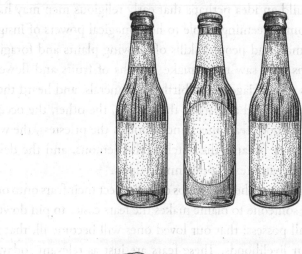

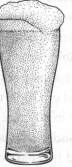
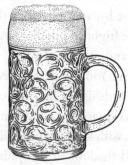

DARK MAGIC

As the earliest agriculturalists, women observed the course of the seasons and weather and many would become skilled in predicting their course and patterns. The superstition that witches could raise a storm was far more likely to be their real ability to predict one (and these superstitions were no doubt taken advantage of by a few opportunistic cunning folks who were only too happy to sell 'fair winds' to sailors in the forms of charms and knotted ropes). To foresee forthcoming changes, whether that be weather, season, or family fortunes and health, was a practised skill. So, what appeared to many to be magic – that witches could create thunder or storms at will, or create illness – was much more likely to be skills in prediction, one they would then be subject to be blamed for.

You can begin to build an idea perhaps that early religious men may have looked upon these women seemingly able to hold magical powers of insight over the weather, animals and people, skills of growing plants and foraging in woodlands. Perhaps they saw them make wreaths of fruits and flowers, partake in group rites of marriages, childbirth and funerals, and heard them speak of spirits of the land and ancestors: the unseen, the other, the occult. Through that lens of religion, fear, anger and jealousy, the priestess, the wise men and cunning women became the witches, the demons, and the devils that feature so vividly in early texts condemning them.

Projected fear plays a big part here – groups often project their fears onto others. Somehow, having someone to blame makes the fears easier to pin down.

There are fears we all possess: that our loved ones will become ill, that we may lose them, or our livelihoods. These fears are just as relevant today as in times gone by, and for many, the witch was somewhere to project all that fear into one frightful bundle, often portrayed as barely human, just a ball of evil actions and malicious intent, so one could feel no guilt in torturing and burning them. You can perhaps even see the appeal of trying to destroy fears and all the hardships of life, misfortune, and evil in its many forms.

The witch's image changes from country to country, from community to community, with local concepts of witches and witchcraft morphing to reflect the fears and shadows of a population. And it could even boost community spirit, as a group's collective shadows are bundled up and cast out with one witch. Witch accusers thought themselves noble and 'righteous' and it may well have been a cause for celebration as a poor rural village burns a witch, believing her to be the reason all their crops failed... Sadly, it would take many centuries from the beginning of Europe's witch hunts for people to realize that burning a witch does nothing to improve weather, crops or food yields.

With the arrival of the printing press in the 1400s, many of these fears, superstitions, ideas and biases were spread widely as fact. The idea of demonic forces empowering the acts of *maleficium*[*] gave the term "witch" new connotations of evil and heresy, and the very real threat of dangerous women.

Books like *Fortalitium Fidei* and *Formicarius,* both written in the mid-1400s, *Malleus Maleficarum* (1487) and *On Witches and Female Soothsayers* (1489) along with pamphlets printed documenting witch trials, were all part of the movement to transform the idea of magic as the practice of beliefs and rituals to its more modern perception of witchcraft, which was that of destructive magic, demonic gatherings and conspiracy. Magic, heresy, and the folkloric night-flight were all brought together, and magic became associated with a new and terrible idea of witchcraft, where fear around magical practices became commonplace, and a distrust of women grew.

OTHERNESS

Why does the witch both terrify and enthral us so?

Witches represent a shadow embodied: the witch can be everything that we as humans are, but wish we weren't...or aren't but wish we were – and that can stir up negative emotions and reactions. It's an uncomfortable truth that all people have the potential to do harm, and oh, how much easier life would be if all the 'baddies' were as easily identified as green-skinned fairytale witches with black hats on a broomstick or a horned devil.

And so the witch becomes a cipher for otherness. Otherness is a waymarker of how we can define ourselves, so if we consider ourselves 'good', the 'other' might be viewed as 'bad.' The stereotypical 'bad' witch is (amongst other things) greedy, cruel, angry, clever, scheming, anti-social, selfish, rude, scary perhaps – embodying the collective shadow self of our society.

---

[*]   A commonly used Latin term at the time, referring to witchcraft and magical acts which harmed people or property.

"Othering" is perhaps one of the most significant obstacles to diverse humans living in harmony and understanding. It has given rise to many prejudices and persecutions over the course of history, including *ethnocentrism,* a belief that the way we do things is natural and right. In contrast, the way others do things is strange, unnatural, or wrong.

For a time in classical society, Christianity and paganism may have existed in harmony, but Christianity, at some point, began looking upon these 'old ways' as rivals, others. This, combined with a worldview dominated by reason would, in time, undermine ancient magical and mystical perceptions of life. Magical thinking is, in a sense, primal, primitive, a word that is painted to be derogatory by religious and scientific schools of thought. And the healer, the cunning one, the priestess became the prototype of the witch destined to burn. Previously accepted womanly skills were now dismissed. Healing practices were pushed into the shadows, which led towards a domain of secrecy, and women were accused of occult and esoteric practices. Sorceress, midwife, herbalist, priestess and witch: all these figures were and are vibrant reflections of (a predominantly) female culture and history – cast into shadow.

CURSED COOKING

As we have seen, witchcraft and cooking have always been intertwined. And in turn, women, cooking and the domestic realm have long been implicated in the paranoia of the existence of evil witch figures. Accusations of poisoned food were part of the subversion of nurturers and women. And places around the home also became part of the stories, myths and witchcraft cases, referring to places we may traditionally define as feminine spaces: the home and specifically the kitchen.

Accusations often mirrored the direct opposite of what women were actually doing: a distortion of their roles and skills in the domestic environment. The act of feeding became accusations of poisoning; child-rearing became eating and killing babies; healing became harming; giving birth became murder and inducing death; and farm work became destroying crops and souring milk, rather than creating things like butter, cheese and other foods.

Women were in a position of some power through the rearing of children and feeding of the household. The witchcraft persecutions could definitely be viewed as part of a distrust of any power held by women – even the modest (but essential) rule of the home. Resulting in bids to control and assert patriarchal power. Sowing seeds of suspicion that would involve both accusing women and turning women against each other as well. Lines blurred in people's minds, between having the skill to cut up and roast a carcass or kill and skin a hare and using that skill to injure others.

It seems that almost any skill or possession or characteristic could be turned into the mark of a witch. The notorious Witchfinder General published a book in 1647 that features an illustration showing the kinds of 'familiars' that witches were thought to call forth to assist their wicked spells. (In England, confessions often focused on relations between the accused and a small animal – a mouse, a toad, a fly, a cat – which fed off the witch's blood: this creature was called a familiar.) And many of the animals have names that evoke echoes of the kitchen craft of their owners: Vinegar Tom; Sacke* and Sugar, and Pyewackett† and Griezzell Greedigut all feature in the illustration. The nurturing nature of these women extended to caring for these animals, but that also made them targets for witch accusations. The simple act of caring for animals or keeping animals to chase mice or guard livestock was, once again, twisted and distorted into some kind of evil act.

COOKING UP A STORM

When you go through all the implements witches were said to fly on: pestle and mortar, cauldron, oven forks, barrels, mops, spoons, as well as broomsticks,‡ we are also seeing a list of kitchen tools. The witch was persistently connected to the kitchen through her instruments.

Sieves are another kitchen tool mentioned as modes of travel for witches. In the North Berwick witch trials, a group of women was famously accused of plotting to raise a storm to sink the ship of King James and his new bride. One of the women, a folk healer called Agnes Sampson, confessed that upon

---

* Another word for wine.
† Pye is an archaic spelling of pie.
‡ Flight on brooms was particular to central European ideas. English witches were more likely to travel in the form of animals, fly without brooms or just walk! But the broom has still become a stereotype the world over.

the night of Halloween she, and some two hundred other witches gathered together went to the sea, "each one in a riddle or sieve" with great flagons of wine and having a merry old time on the way.

And when it came to setting sail into the ocean another very popular method was via shell: witches were known to "saile in an egge shell, a cockle or mussel shell, through and under the tempestuous seas."[+] Because witches could sail in eggshells, it became common practice in the British Isles and Europe to crush eggshells or poke them full of holes, to prevent witches or fairies setting to sea in them, raising storms and wrecking ships. Or, as some witches from Norfolk were said to do, drown sailors by stirring up eggshells in pails of water, creating a tiny storm in buckets to raise storms at sea.

But witches can also use eggshells for good, as this little story tells.

The Gypsy Girl and The Grateful Witch

From a version found in Gypsy Sorcery and Fortune Telling, *by Charles Godfrey Leland (1891).*

Once there was a gypsy girl who noticed that when anybody ate eggs, they broke up the shells. When she asked why, she received this answer:

You must break the shell to bits for fear
Lest the witches should make it a boat, my dear.
For over the sea away from home,
Far by night, the witches roam.

"I don't see why the poor witches should not have boats as well as other people", she said, and threw the shell of an egg which she had been eating as far as she could, crying, *"Chovihani, lav tro bero!"* ("Witch – there is your boat!") and to her amazement the little shell was caught up by the wind and whirled away, and a voice cried, *"Paraka!"* ("I thank you!")

Now, it came to pass some time later that the gypsy girl was caught in a great flood, trapped on a small piece of land. The water rose higher and higher, and the girl was sure she would drown. But, just in time, she saw a woman in a white boat. A woman with witches' eyes. She was rowing the boat with a broom, and a black cat sat on her shoulder. "Jump in!" she cried to the girl and then rowed her to dry land.

When she was on the shore, the woman said, "Turn round three times to the right and look each time at the boat." As the girl did so, each time she turned and looked, she saw the boat grow smaller and smaller, until... it was as an eggshell.

And the woman sang:

That is the shell you threw to me,
Even a witch can grateful be.

And with a smile, she vanished: cat, broom, shell, and all.

Witches and fairies were also said to ride on items you might find in the field or garden – straw, bullrushes, ragwort, cabbage stalks, fern roots, and other types of grass were steeds that could carry them through the air. Ragwort earned its folk name "fairy horse" in this way. The fairies may "steal hempen stalks from the fields where they grow, to convert them into horses."⁵ Isobel Gowdie, on trial for witchcraft in 1662, said that when people saw bits of corn straw flying in the air on warm breezes it was actually witches travelling – inspired, perhaps, by the way straw can whirl in the wind and seeing magic within it. Swirls of leaves are still said, in Celtic cultures, to be evidence of fairies. The tiniest of fairies are believed to ride on falling leaves, and if a leaf is caught in the air, before it has touched the ground, the fairy must grant you a wish.

Talk of enchantment, flight and travel are words that can be interpreted in more than one way. From the visions of both accused witches and supposed victims, we could conjecture many ideas of hallucinations, dreams, shamanistic journeying, trance states. But also possibly of depression, anxiety and neurodiversity, and seeing the world in different ways, many variables which could play a part in the ideas of witches and devils.

Many witches' kitchens would have contained items that could, used improperly, be poisons – belladonna (deadly nightshade), yew and very possibly

substances of hallucinatory and psychotropic nature: certain mushrooms, mugwort, henbane and applethorn (also known as devil's snare). These herbs could
have produced feelings of flight, of leaving one's body and astral travel. These
could have been used for a selection of reasons – as they are now – for healing
mental health issues, spiritual journeying, meditation, and recreational use.

*For the most skillful among the witches could cause themselves to fall into
the Witches' Sleep, as they called this trance, whenever they chose; others
had to submit to tedious and often abominable ceremonies…thus it was
well known that certain herbs, like aconite, produce in sleep the sensation
of flying, and they were, of course, diligently employed. Hyosciamus* and
taxus†, hypericum‡ and asafoetida§ were great favourites.*[6]

Hallucinogenic plants and tinctures made in the kitchen of the witch may
well have been a way for people to 'journey' and 'fly' in a spiritual sense like
the oracle or shaman seeks other realms of consciousness, and altered mental
states to help divination and seeing. But it may also have been an escape from
oppressive environments: even to dance around the fire and keen and sing
would be a freedom for many.

Whatever the truth of it, the image of the broomstick and the applying
of ointments to oneself or the broom stick really stuck in imaginations, and
as rumour carried that witches could fly, their prosecutors used this myth
to suggest that witches were dealing with dark forces – and punished them
accordingly.

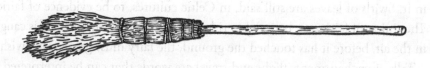

---

*   Also known as henbane.
†   Yew.
‡   St John's Wort.
§   A kind of giant fennel often used to replace onion and garlic in cookery.

SECTION ONE SUMMARY

KITCHEN WITCHES TODAY

There are goddesses of the kitchen, fat and happy, dwelling above the extractor fan, or just behind the Tate and Lyle cans. Give them good greeting, and count yourself amongst them.

Alice Tarbuck, from an article on dangerouswomenproject.org about the Kitchen Witch (2016)

I do not believe that any of the people killed in the witch hunts were witches in the way that their accusers saw them, as in the demonic, flying, baby boilin', storm raisin', monstrous hags created as superstition. They were innocent of being these witches of fiction and more likely persecuted for who they were and not what they had done. As current-day campaigners for pardons for these men and women remind us, in any court of law today, they would be innocent because not one shred of true evidence existed for the crime of witchcraft: it was hearsay, superstitions, completely false ideas such as witch's marks, familiars and witch pricking, and of course, testimonies drawn out from fear, bullying, torture, leading questions, months of imprisonment and awful treatment.

I do believe that many of the accused were, however, witches as we use the word today: people skilled with herbs, potions, spells and similar crafts, keepers of stories, of pagan practices and celebrations. Knowledge of plant and herb healing magic may have bubbled in their sacred cauldrons, and a rare few may have even used this knowledge for truly nefarious purposes. I do believe not one of them deserved the treatment and torture they received: their knowledge was earned through a lifetime of quietly and steadfastly feeding and fuelling those around them. Many had gifts of everyday magic: the knowledge of how to feed and heal themselves and others from the earth, skills we now barely register as something of importance, much perhaps, like the historical work of women in the kitchen.

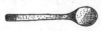

Visioning the Modern Witch

Witch as a word has spent many centuries intended purely as an insult or accusation, a label few, if anyone, wanted. But witch, both the name and figure, is being reclaimed, and reworked by many. It is being built upon with new names: Green Witch, Sea Witch, Hearth Witch, Kitchen Witch are part of that creation of positivity around the word witch. And similarly, witchcraft, as we may call it today, is being fully recognised as a tradition rooted in folk magic and a patchwork of older magical practices, paganism and mythology. For many, claiming the title witch is about reclaiming ancestral knowledge, skills and intuition. The name of the Kitchen Witch is steeped in exciting and ancient history. Kitchen witchery can feel like returning to the roots of witchcraft, back when women and men practiced witchcraft at their hearth fires in ancient dwellings for connection and insight.

Pasta

I assign them to their fate.
Silent, unbending, anonymous.
Thrust upright into the bubbling cauldron,
They stand a few minutes.
I watch their mute surrender
As they bow away under the steam.
Submerging the last unyielding bits,
I am the Kitchen Witch;
Doing nothing
And dreaming of power.

Deborah Joyce (1990)

Stories of the witch are drawn through history. Actually, dragged, might be a better word, as she picks up new scraps of stories as she goes, like twigs in tangled hair. From the civilisations of Greece and Rome, all the way up to the present day, ideas and stereotypes draw from vast reservoirs of history, myth, folklore and superstition. How do you walk a joyful path from such a challenging history? Can we turn this language, these stereotypes around?

As we as a society change, our witches and stories can change too, not to erase the past but build from it. Turning away from old stories from men who feared powerful women in Judeo-Christian religions and reclaiming some of the traditions that were cast into shadow and demonised. And though not everyone is happy that witchcraft has become so trendy that any high-street shop may now contain books on basic spells and herbs, perhaps this is a return to when magic and its craft were simply part of everyday life. Life in centuries past was incredibly hard, cruel, challenging and unpredictable, and maybe the witches of that era reflected that. Now, perhaps, a freedom is afforded to us to allow our witches to be lighter, brighter. Maybe this is the witch we need now. Maybe, after all we've been through, we can fear the witch less and connect to her more.

Drawing pagan rituals into the present can hold paradoxes, as we may no longer fear spirits or gods as governing our survival in the same way. And it's obviously no longer appropriate to sacrifice animals – so yes, we are pulling on what you might call the 'nicer' elements of ritual and ceremony, if we are recreating these practices today. That's not necessarily a bad thing. We live in very different times, with far more security of health, food and shelter. But perhaps in everyday life, we are lacking in other areas like empathy, mindful awareness and connection to nature. The magic of every culture and era reflects what is needed, so perhaps we need more comfort, kindness, compassion and connection.

We have the freedom to embrace new ideas of the witch as a pathway to possibilities. Witchcraft is not, however, all cosy and lovely, there is both light and dark. It can be a route for many to connect to grief, sorrow and anger. Your rituals may involve working through feelings of remorse, guilt and regret like at the *deipnon* for Hecate. So, if to be a witch is a path you seek, remember the history upon which you walk, respect it, and take joy that this way is here for you. You have every right to occupy it, but do show it, and our forewitches respect and humility. To call yourself a witch is to be part of a legacy. A lineage of the wyrd and the wise, those who walked (and flew) before us. It won't always be easy, but it can gift us space to address our fears, anxieties, anger, and power.

Becoming More Ourselves

What does cookery mean? It means the knowledge of Medea and of Circe, and of Calypso, and Sheba. It means knowledge of all herbs, and fruits, and balms and spices... It means the economy of your great-grandmother and the science of modern chemistry, and French art, and Arabian hospitality. It means, in fine, that you are to see imperatively that everyone has something nice to eat.

John Ruskin (1819-1900)

I believe Kitchen Witchery and food magic is so appealing to us today, among other reasons, because it feels, for many, like the hearth fire and kitchen itself: welcoming, inviting and enveloping, a place of memory, warmth, candlelight and smoke. This is coming home to the world of magic and wise women.

And when we speak of the accused witches of the past, we mourn them, we marvel at what they endured and feel regret that they had to. But also, don't forget that they had great skill and knowledge. Everyone – from those who never performed a spell to those who perhaps did consider themselves witches, the quiet wives, the outsiders and the oddballs. They were powerful for simply being women, for being wise ones, for being fairy witches, for trying to help, even for being the village scold or nagging wife that had no time or inclination to be polite in society. They stood out for all manner of reasons; they suffered and died for all manner of reasons – for being notable enough to be singled out by townsfolk. Perhaps learning from them is our best way to honour them, understand as best we can, and do our best not to let history repeat itself.

Maybe the witch to you represents a lavish going-against the norms, crossing boundaries, voicing one's opinions, drinking, cackling loudly, making noise, taking up space, feasting and dancing. Maybe it means a lack of guilt or shame, finding meaning in a spiritual landscape without the disempowerment or subjugation of many mainstream religions. That one should feel guilt for one's pleasures is something the witch has perhaps always rejected as an idea, in both fairy tales and 'real life.' Those who were opinionated, who earned their own money or owned their own land, maybe they didn't fit into the flow of society. And maybe you don't have to either.

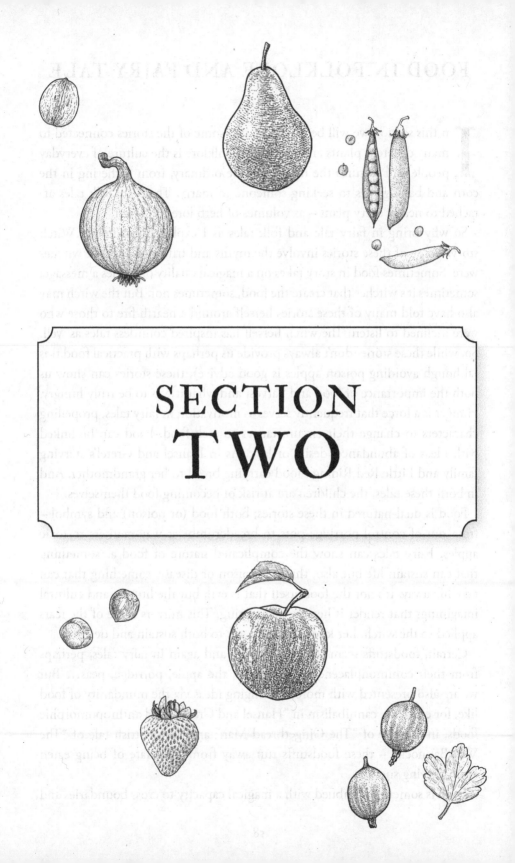

SECTION TWO

FOOD IN FOLKLORE AND FAIRY TALE

I n this section we will be exploring just some of the stories connected to many different plants and foodstuffs. Folklore is the culture of everyday people and features the mundane, the ordinary, from gathering in the corn and baking pies to seeking someone to marry. There are folk tales attached to nearly every plant – as volumes of herb lore can attest.

So why bring in fairy tale and folk tales as I explore the Kitchen Witch story? Some of these stories involve the myths and truths of who the witches were. Sometimes food in story takes on a magical quality or carries a message, sometimes it's witches that create the food, sometimes not. But the witch may also have told many of these stories herself around a hearth fire to those who were inclined to listen. The witch herself has inspired countless tales as well. So, while these stories don't always provide us perhaps with practical food tips (although avoiding poison apples is good advice), these stories can show us both the importance of food and harvest and what it was to be truly hungry. Hunger is a force that frequently serves as motivation in fairy tales, propelling characters to change their circumstances to seek food. Food can be linked with ideas of abundance, desire or lack. As in Hansel and Gretel's starving family and Little Red Riding Hood carrying bread to her grandmother. And in both these tales, the children are at risk of becoming food themselves.

Food is dual-natured in these stories; both food (or poison) and symbol – from out-of-control porridge pots to breadcrumbs as way-markers to toxic apples. Fairy tales can show the complicated nature of food as something that can sustain life but also, through poison or disease, something that can take life away. It's not the food itself that is evil, but the human and cultural imaginings that render it healing or harming. This mirrors some of the fears applied to the witch: her knowledge is a gift to both sustain and destroy.

Certain foodstuffs seem to pop up again and again in fairy tales, perhaps from their commonplaceness: the walnut, the apple, porridge, peas... But we are also presented with more challenging ideas via the mundanity of food like, for example, cannibalism in "Hansel and Gretel," and anthropomorphic foods, in the tale of "The Gingerbread Man" and the Scottish tale of "The Wee Bannock" – these foodstuffs run away from their fate of being eaten (with varying success).

Food is sometimes imbued with a magical capacity to cross boundaries and hold transformative powers, it may be infused with magic or used as a tool or test of some kind. With the Greek myth of Persephone it was the pomegranate seeds that changed her, making her part of the Underworld. The poisoned apple transports Snow White into a place between the living and the dead. Eating foods of the fairy folk or fae can connect you to their world, and there are many tales from Scottish witch trials of "Fairy-Witches" – accused witches who claimed to draw their powers from the fairies, feasting and dancing with them and learning their skills.

FOOD, LORE AND CHANGE

Folklore is a story form that can be considered a way to reinterpret the world and our place in it – what we fear and what we cherish – which changes as the world changes. Food possesses forms of magic in fairy tales, to represent and evoke change (powers you may suggest exist in real life too – food can change people in fiction and reality). Food represents change, and often we use food to represent passages of time, marking special occasions with it. But also, food, like life, is impermanent.

Time is precious, as we see in Cinderella's tale written by Charles Perrault, she travels within the pumpkin as her coach, but it has a distinct expiry date (midnight) she must heed.

Hansel and Gretel

"Hansel and Gretel" is a tale of displacement due to food, or lack thereof. Unable to feed them, Hansel and Gretel's parents send them into the forest. They try to use food (breadcrumbs) to guide their way back home. When they come across a house of bread with sugared windows, they delight in feasting in abundance: they are saved! But then, the children become potential food themselves, and the witch's house becomes a prison. In the end, the witch becomes a human sacrifice in exchange for the riches that Hansel and Gretel take from her.

A poor woodcutter and his wife lived on the edge of a large forest. He could barely provide the daily bread for his wife and two children, Hansel and Gretel. One night his wife said to him, "We must take the children into the middle of the forest and leave them there. We can no longer feed them, if we don't, we shall all starve."

The children, still awake, heard everything that their mother said. Gretel began to cry. But Hansel whispered, "Don't cry. I'll find a way to help us," and he got up and crept outside. Under the moonlight, he gathered as many white pebbles from the ground as he could. Early the next morning, before sunrise, they set out.

When they reached the heart of the forest, they lit a fire. Their mother said, "Now, children, rest by the fire, we're going into the forest to gather wood. We'll come back and get you." Hansel and Gretel sat by the fire waiting for their mother and father to return. Night fell, and the full moon rose, Hansel took Gretel by the hand. The pebbles glittered like silver coins and showed them the way home. They walked the whole night long and were back at their house by dawn.

Their father rejoiced when he saw his children again. But not long after this, there was, once again, nothing to eat in the house. And come dawn, once more, they found themselves walking into the forest. All Hansel had this time was a little bread, which he scattered on the ground as he had the pebbles. The children were led even deeper into the forest, and once again, they were to sleep by the fire, and once again, their parents did not return. Gretel shared her bread with Hansel because he had dropped his along the path.

When the moon rose, Hansel looked for the breadcrumbs. But they were gone. The birds had gobbled them up. The children soon lost their way amongst the trees, walking all night, and all day until they fell asleep from exhaustion. They were now also very hungry. But as luck would have it, they came to a little house made of bread, with cake for roof tiles and clear sugar panes for windows.

Hansel had eaten a good piece of roof, and Gretel had devoured several small round windows before they heard a shrill voice cry from inside: "Nibble, Nibble, I hear a mouse! Who's that nibbling on my house?" Hansel and Gretel were so frightened they dropped their handfuls of the house.

A small, old woman appeared at the door. "Well now, dear children, where did you come from? Come inside with me." She made them a meal of milk and pancakes with sweet fruits and nuts. Afterwards, she made up two soft beds, and Hansel and Gretel thought themselves in heaven. The hag, however, was really a wicked witch. She had built the house only to lure children to her so she could kill, cook, and eat them. It would be a happy feast day for her.

Early the next morning, she grabbed Hansel and stuck him into a cage. She shook Gretel and sent her to fetch water and cook breakfast, so that they may fatten up Hansel for eating. Frightened, Gretel did as the Witch demanded.

Time passed and one evening, the Witch declared today would be the day that Hansel would be cooked. But first they would bake some bread, a nice fresh loaf to accompany the main course. The old woman's eyes were weak, so she called Gretel over to see if the bread was cooked. "Sit down on the board," she said, "and I'll shove you inside so that you can look properly."

The Witch planned to trap Gretel inside, to bake and eat her too, of course. But Gretel was clever and said, "Show me how. Sit down on the board, and I'll shove you inside." And as the old woman sat on the board, Gretel shoved her inside as far as she could, and shut the oven door and bolted it shut. The old woman screamed in the hot oven, and Gretel ran off and freed Hansel as the Witch burned to death.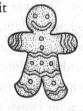

They filled their pockets with sweets and valuables from the cottage and found their way home. Their father rejoiced to see them again. His wife had died, and apparently, he hadn't spent a single happy day since his children had been away. Now he was a rich man.

Fruit appears in myths around the world as a symbol of abundance, associated with goddesses of fertility and the harvest, whilst specific kinds of fruit have acquired their own symbolic meanings in the myths and legends of different cultures. Fruits and their stories have travelled the globe with explorers, traders and settlers to be cultivated in new lands. For many ancient people, before being introduced to such enchanting delights as chocolate and sugar cane (or unable to afford them), fruits were, along with honey and sweet nuts, the pinnacle of sweet decadence for millennia. This is often reflected in the stories of golden goddesses, temptation, abundance, and revelry.

Apples

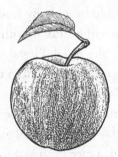

I am the ancient apple-queen,
As once I was, so am I now.
For evermore a hope unseen,
Betwixt the blossom and the bough...

William Morris, "Pomona" (1891)

Crisp, sweet and juicy, apples are one of the most prevalent fruits found in myth and fairy tale from ancient times onwards in Europe and the Middle East. They are rich with symbolic meanings and mythical associations, including wisdom, immortality, resurrection, knowledge, and fertility. Apples are often associated with female deities like Pomona, the Roman goddess and guardian of flourishing fruit trees – shiny apples and juicy pears, gardens, and orchards. In artworks we often see her with arms filled with fruit and wearing an apple crown making sure all around her bloom and thrive. But those apples are so appealing, sometimes they get stolen...

Stolen Gold...

In Greek myth, the Earth Mother, Gaia, gifts Hera, Queen of the gods, precious apple trees that fruit golden apples which taste of honey and hold magical healing properties. The trees are guarded by a fierce dragon and tended by the Hesperides, daughters of the evening. Each evening, the golden apples cast their radiant glow across the sky creating the golden colours of the sunset.

For one of his twelve great labours, the hero Hercules had to obtain some of these apples. He enlists the help of the giant, Atlas, who kills the dragon and collects the fruits. Hercules then takes the apples to Greece, but Athena returns them to the Hesperides.

In another tale of these golden apples, a goddess manages not only to procure one, but to set in motion the events that cause the Trojan War, one of the key events in Greek mythology. The story goes that the goddess of discord, Eris, is angry that she has not been invited to attend a wedding feast. And so, arriving uninvited, she throws a single golden apple, with the label "For the Fairest" onto a table. Hera, Athena, and Aphrodite each assume that the apple was meant for themselves. They ask Paris, Prince of Troy, to settle the matter, and he awards the apple to Aphrodite. In revenge, Hera and Athena support the war and the fall of Troy, an episode that is also known as the Judgement of Paris. The term "apple of discord" is still used to refer to something that provokes an argument. (Note the whispers of "fairest of them all" and the uninvited guest causing trouble – we'll see these themes in the fairy stories of Snow White and Sleeping Beauty many centuries later.)

Another mythical story of goddesses and golden apples comes from Iceland and is shared in the *Eddas* (medieval works of Icelandic and Norse folklore). It features Idunn, the goddess of Norse mythology, keeper of the golden apples of youth, which are very precious, as even the gods would grow old without them. In this story, the trickster god Loki gets himself into a quarrel with a giant and promises to kidnap Idunn and give her to the giant to placate him. He lures Idunn out of Asgard, the home of the gods, and into a wood, with the promise of interesting apples. The giant snatches Idunn from the forest and takes her to his home. But Idunn's absence causes the gods to grow old and grey, and they are furious when they find that Loki is responsible for her absence. Loki promises to return her, and he borrows Freya's magic cloak, which turns him into a falcon. He turns Idunn into a hazelnut and in their disguises he is able to take her safely back to Asgard.

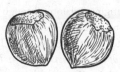

Deceptive apples...

A theme we have seen more than once in stories is apples used for deception, the apple being a symbol for earthly pleasures, gluttony, and temptation. Early examples include the Bible's creation myth, in Genesis, where Eve eats the fruit of the Tree of Knowledge. It's not stated what this fruit actually is, but the apple is a popular interpretation[*]. In eating the fruit, Eve is banished from the Garden of Eden and she and all women for eternity are cursed with the pain of childbirth as punishment for her disobedience.

In the story of Snow White it is an apple once again that delivers a curse. In The Brothers Grimm version of the tale, the jealous Queen orders that Snow White's lungs and liver are retrieved for her to cook and eat with salt – something of the cannibal witch archetype there. But when Snow White escapes this fate, a poisoned apple is employed. Half of this apple is green and good, half is red and poisoned. The Queen bites into the green half, thus convincing Snow White that the apple is safe to eat. But in consuming the poisoned section, Snow White dies and lies in a glass coffin until rescued by a prince. In Grimm's first edition,[†] the ending is a little different to the one we may know now: the prince, so enamoured with Snow White's corpse, keeps her in the coffin near him always, and only eats when he is stood in front of it. His servants, who tire of carrying the coffin, take her out and inadvertently dislodge the apple stuck in her throat, bringing her back to life.

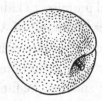

Somerset Apples (and other feasts)
– My local witches

Accounts of my 'local witches' at the Somerset witch trials around the 1660s can be found in a book called *Saducismus Triumphatus, or, Full and plain evidence concerning witches and apparitions* written by Joseph Glanvill, a writer, clergyman, and rector of Bath Abbey. The book was published posthumously in 1681 and was based on original records made by magistrate Robert Hunt and a collection of earlier works by Glanvill. The work is considered notable in detailing the accounts of the Somerset trials of 1657-1665 (though as always biases and inaccuracies are suggested, we work with what we have). These trials are obviously interesting to me as this is my local area, but also these are some of the more detailed of the English cases when it comes to food.

The trials of these accused witches, including Alice Duke, Elizabeth Style, Jane Brooks and Anne Bishop, not only present a rather jolly account of food and feasting, but also a suggestion that for some, these revels were something of a joyful escape (whether they were imagined in vision or happened in real life, we don't know).

Elizabeth Style said that the Devil,

Promised her Mony, and that she should live gallantly, and have the pleasure of the world for Twelve years, if she would with her blood sign his Paper, which was to give her soul to him. […] Then they [the Devil and her fellow witches] *did drink Wine, and eat Cakes and Meat.*[‡]

Alice Duke gave a similar account:

At their meeting they have usually Wine or good Beer, Cakes, Meat or the like. They eat and drink really when they meet in their bodies, dance also and have Musick...

At parting they cried: *Merry meet, merry part!* a greeting and farewell still used today by modern-day witches.

[‡]   It's not easy at some points in the source material to untangle who said what. This is what I believe is being said and it seems that both Duke and Style were asked very similar, and possibly leading, questions.

I mention my local witches here because the trial records hold more than one story of poison apples, which perhaps is no surprise as apples continue to be a very popular crop in Somerset, earning it the epithet of "cider country." These stories also have more than a whisper of fairy tale about them. Both Elizabeth Style and Jane Brooks offered up apples to people, who would later accuse them of *maleficium*.

Elizabeth, in one account, brings two apples to the house of a woman called Agnes, and offers up "one of them a very fair red Apple, which Style desired her to eat, which she did, and in a few hours was taken ill and worse than ever she had been before…" Agnes claimed herself "bewitched" and died not long after. In a separate event, Jane Brooks offered apples to a boy in return for bread, after he takes the apple he falls ill, but he survived the ordeal.

In another book that draws on the accounts recorded by Hunt and Glanvill I think this assessment of the accounts of witches meetings in Somerset really sums up the witch trial disconnect of the rumours and superstitions, and what the women were actually doing, pretty succinctly:

> *Even in the Somerset case, in which the suspected witches admitted to attending an outdoor meeting and worshipping the devil, seems to have been pretty tame by comparison to the popular portrayal of such scenes. There were no sacrifices of babies or wild orgiastic scenes. Instead, English witches between 1640 and 1670 seemed content to stick some thorns into some wax dolls and sit down to a meal of beef and beer.*

> Frederick Valletta, *Witchcraft, Magic and Superstition in England 1640–70*

There is a wealth of folklore using apples to see the future, specifically on special festival days – you'll see more of divination with apples in Section Four at Samhain. But for now, let's see how Baba Yaga imparts apple-lore.

The Silver Saucer and the Red Apple
– A Russian Fairy Tale

Adapted from Russian Fairy Tales *by Moura Budberg (1965). The author of this collection of fairy tales was herself every bit as fascinating as Baba Yaga, as a baroness, adventuress, suspected double-agent and spy!*

In other versions of this tale, the apple is made of crystal, which is a beautiful image, but I liked this version as the red apple, like in Snow White and the Somerset witch trials, is suggestive of a little bewitchment afoot…

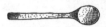

Once upon a time there lived in a small village, a peasant and his wife, who had three daughters. The two elder daughters were lazy and vain, but the youngest, Aliona, was modest and kind. She worked hard, cleaning and cooking, weeding the vegetable garden, and drawing the water.

One day an old woman, Baba Yaga, came up to the house and begged for a piece of bread to soothe her hunger. The elder girls would not speak to her, but Aliona gave her a nice fat potato cake. "Thank you, my girl," the old woman said. "In return for your kindness, I will give you a sweet crumb of advice. When your father goes to the fair and asks what you would like him to bring you, ask him to buy you a silver saucer and a red apple. When you have them, roll the apple on the saucer and say:

Roll apple, roll
On the silver saucer
Show me on the saucer
The cities and the fields
The forests and the seas
And the tall mountains
And the beauty of the skies.

"And should you ever be in trouble, my girl, you can count on me. Remember: I live on the edge of a dark forest and it takes exactly three days and three nights to get to my home."

Soon after this day, the father decided to go to the fair. He asked his daughters what they should like him to bring them back. One daughter asked for bright cotton cloth for a dress, the other asked for patterned silk. But Aliona asked, as advised, for a silver saucer and a red apple. When he returned, he brought the present for his daughters: bright cotton and patterned silk, and a silver saucer and red apple for Aliona. The elder girls gloated over their presents and laughed at Aliona, wondering what she would do with a silver saucer and an apple. Aliona did not eat the apple, much as she wanted to – instead, she sat down in a corner, and rolled it on the saucer and whispered to it the words the old woman had told her:

Roll apple, roll
On the silver saucer
Show me on the saucer
The cities and the fields
The forests and the seas
And the tall mountains
And the beauty of the skies.

And behold, there in the saucer could be seen great cities, villages nestling in the fields, ships on the seas, the high mountains and the blue skies, the bright sun and the pale moon were there too, with the stars chasing one another…all so beautiful you couldn't describe it, even in fairy tale…

The sisters gazed at the scene with envy and tried to tempt Aliona into exchanging the saucer and the apple for the presents their father had brought them. But nothing would persuade her to part with her treasures. They decided to get the saucer and the apple by fair means or foul.

"Darling Aliona," they whispered, "let us go to the wood and gather strawberries."

Aliona gave the saucer and the apple to her father and went to the wood with her sisters. She walked and walked, gathering strawberries all the way, and the sisters enticed her farther and farther on. When she was deep in the heart of the wood, they sprang upon her and buried her under a birch tree.[*] When they came home at night they said Aliona had run away and disappeared, that the wolves must have caught her. Their father and mother

---

[*]   In Celtic mythology, the birch tree is a symbol of renewal. In Russian folklore they were considered magical and a symbol of the feminine; pagan Russians might touch a birch tree for good luck.

wept bitterly. The sisters simply kept asking their father to give them the saucer and the apple. But he refused, putting them into a locked chest.

One day, not long after, a shepherd was following his flock through the wood, and deep in the heart of the wood, he saw a graceful white birch tree and under it a mound with red and blue flowers growing over it and reeds swaying above it. He cut off a reed and made a pipe, and – oh what magic! – the pipe began to sing all by itself:

Play, play, little shepherd,
Play softly,
Play gently,
Alas, I was killed
And buried under the birch tree
For the sake of the silver saucer,
For the sake of the red apple.

The shepherd came to the village, and the pipe went on singing. The people gathered around to listen. Aliona's parents happened to be passing by, and they heard the song and it pained their hearts.

They asked the shepherd to show them the spot where he found the reed, and they followed him to the forest. They found the mound with the red and blue flowers and dug it up, and there lay Aliona. They recognised their favourite daughter and wept bitter tears over her.

The father took the reed pipe, and it began to sing:

Play, play, Father dear,
Play softly,
Play gently,
My sisters lured me into the forest
And killed me there
And buried me under the birch tree
All to get the silver saucer
And to get the red apple.
Go now through the forest, Father dear,
Far, far, to the other end of the forest,
Where you will find a thatched cottage
And a kind old woman is living in it.

She will give you some fresh water in a jar.
Sprinkle me with it
And I will wake from this heavy slumber,
From this sleep of death.

The father and mother went to the other end of the forest to the little hut. An old woman came out on the porch, and they asked her for some fresh water as the song had instructed.

"I will help Aliona," the old woman replied, "because she has a kind heart." She gave them a jar of water. The parents thanked the old woman and started on the homeward journey. They gathered the wicked sisters from their home, along with the shepherd and a crowd from the village, all seeking to watch this strange tale unfold. They made their way to the birch tree in the forest. The father sprinkled his daughter with the water, and Aliona came to life. The wicked sisters' faces turned ashen and they confessed their sins. The village people seized them and banished them forever from their native land. Aliona returned home to live with her parents, and they loved her more than ever before.

Figs

Soft-fleshed and fragrant, the fig is another contender for the fruit that appears in the Garden of Eden. Some artworks depict a fig as the forbidden fruit, and after eating, Adam and Eve cover their nakedness with fig leaves.

In Greek mythology it is Demeter who gifts the fig tree to the mortal realm to repay the hospitality of a king, after he gave her shelter whilst she tried to find her kidnapped daughter, Persephone. Figs are also often associated with Dionysus – Bacchus to the Romans – as god of the grape-harvest, winemaking and wine, fertility, fruit, vegetation, as well as insanity, ritual madness, religious ecstasy, festivity and theatre (so that's everything needed for a good party!). Offerings for Dionysus can include garlands of figs and grape vines, these were also used in festivities in his honour.

In Roman myth the fig tree is a symbol of sovereignty. In the story of Romulus and Remus – the infants that would go on to found the nation of

Rome – they were sheltered under a fig tree after their floating basket got entangled alongside the river in its branches. This is where they were found by the she-wolf that would raise them.

Among the sectors of British culture most influenced by the Romans were agriculture and food. And included in the rich list of crops the Romans introduced here are figs, along with olives, grapes, and herbs including rosemary, bay and fennel.

Gooseberries

Crisp, tart berries, some of the earliest of the season, that grow on prickly bushes, the cultivation of gooseberries was first recorded in England as far back as 1276. This long history of gooseberries in the UK means they have had plenty of time to pick up a great number of local folk names and lore: dayberry, goggle, honey-blob, feaberry, dewberry, wineberry, and gooze-gogs (especially in Somerset – this is what my dad calls them).

If British children ask where babies come from, they might once have been told that they can be found "under a gooseberry bush." This could be connected with the Victorian flower meaning* of the blossom: anticipation.

In the Isle of Wight (a very lovely island off the south coast of England) the Gooseberry Wife was a figure in tales told to children warning that if they went out into the garden, the Gooseberry Wife – portrayed as a large caterpillar – would catch them. The Gooseberry Wife protects the green gooseberries, perhaps making sure they aren't picked too early.

In Germany, gooseberry bushes were planted around cow fields to keep witches out on Walpurgisnacht (more on this celebration later in the book), perhaps because of their thorny branches. As the first fruit of summer, ripening as early as May, gooseberries are popular in the UK at the religious

---

* The language of flowers, also known as floriography, is a means of symbolism and communication through the use of flowers. Its popularity soared in Victorian England, and many books were published during this era. Whilst roses are associated with love and rosemary with remembrance, not all plants had positive connotations, fig for example was connected to arguments, and pomegranates to foolishness. You can read more from classical Victorian era texts on flowers at sentiayoga.com/kitchenwitch

festival of Whitsun (also known as Pentecost) near the end of May. The first gooseberries are often eaten in pies, add that to seasonal milk and cream, and Whitsun feasts would have been quite the treat!

Pumpkin

Earthy and sweet, the bright pumpkin heralds the season of autumn. Pumpkins feature in folklore all around the world: in Indian folktales pumpkins can contain evil spells for safekeeping or protection, and in Chinese lore the pumpkin or gourd is an emblem of abundance, fruitfulness, and good health. And they can grow to such sizes they may have inspired storytellers to think you could travel in one...

Pumpkin Carriages

"Well," said her godmother... *"Run into the garden, and bring me a pumpkin."*

 Cinderella went at once to gather the finest she could get, and brought it to her godmother, not being able to imagine how this pumpkin could help her to go to the ball. Her godmother scooped out all the inside of it, leaving nothing but the rind. Then she struck it with her wand, and the pumpkin was instantly turned into a fine gilded coach.

"Cinderella" or "The Little Glass Slipper", Charles Perrault (1697). Translated by Charles Welsh (1901)

The ram with the golden horns ordered them to bring a coach, and in a moment six goats were seen coming harnessed to a pumpkin of such an enormous size that two persons could sit inside it very comfortably. The pumpkin was dry, and it was lined with soft cushions of down and velvet, and the princess stepped in feeling great admiration for so novel a carriage.

"The Ram" from *Fairy Tales (Les Contes des Fées)* Marie-Catherine d'Aulnoy (1697). Translated by Annie Macdonell and Miss Lee (1892).

Pomegranates

It is great fun to crack open the pithy hull of the pomegranate and release a cascade of juicy little red jewels. The pomegranate has long been a source of food and herbal medicines in the Mediterranean. Its profusion of rosy red seeds made it a symbol of fertility: from one fruit could come many more. It was also connected to marriage, and brides in ancient Rome might be crowned with pomegranate-twig wreaths. In Greece, it was once a custom to throw a pomegranate and break it on the floor before you entered your house for the first time in the New Year to bring good luck. Pomegranate seeds are well known for their appearance in the Greek myth of Persephone.

Persephone and the Pomegranate Seeds

Persephone is picking flowers from a meadow when Hades, rising from the earth, carries her away to be his bride in the Underworld. The goddess Hecate hears the cries of Persephone and tells her mother, Goddess of the Harvest, Demeter, and together they search for her.

Hecate guides Demeter through the dark nights with flaming torches to light her way through many crossroads and paths, but to no avail.

Demeter is so grief-stricken that she casts the earth into barrenness; no crops grow as she mourns. The people of the land are starving, so Persephone's father, the god Zeus, is forced to order Hades to release her from the Underworld.

Hades agrees to let her go, but not before first entreating her to eat some pomegranate seeds. Having consumed food of the Underworld, Persephone becomes part of this realm and must then spend half of each year there, for she is now Queen of the Underworld and a goddess of death. (But still, against her will – the trickery and imprisonment make this a challenging tale to say the least.)

When Persephone returns to her mother each spring, Demeter ensures that the season flourishes, the pomegranate trees blossom and the earth again produces flowers, fruit, and grain. But when autumn falls, Persephone must return to the Underworld. Hecate becomes her companion on her yearly journeys and helps lead her through the realms. And the earth falls into dormancy of the dark winter months as Demeter grieves the loss of her daughter once more.

Pears

Sweet and juicy, pears are sacred to the Greek goddesses Hera, Aphrodite, their Roman counterparts Juno and Venus, along with Pomona, goddess of fruit trees and harvests. We've also seen these goddesses are connected to apples, as the apple and the pear are closely related. In Culpeper's *Complete Herbal*, the pear belongs to Venus, along with the apple and the strawberry. He advises that to boil pears with a little honey creates a potion soothing to an "oppressed stomach."

Pears feature in Homer's *Odyssey* (c. 700 BCE). They were cultivated in Ancient Greece and considered "gifts of the gods" along with apples, pomegranate, figs and olives. Wild pears, like wild apples, can grow thorns for protection, and in Europe, the pear tree was considered a way to protect against evil spirits, so a safeguard pear tree might be planted next to a gate or doorway.

As well as protection, the pear can also represent prosperity and adaptability, as the pear tree has long had a reputation for being able to thrive just about anywhere. After the September 11, 2001 terror attacks at the World Trade Centre in New York, a severely damaged 'survivor tree' was discovered at Ground Zero, with snapped roots and burnt branches. The tree was removed from the rubble and placed into a park where it made a full recovery, new, smooth limbs grew from the gnarled stumps, creating a visible demarcation between the tree's past and present. The tree now stands in a memorial garden: it is a Callery pear tree. This is a wonderful example of how we are adding to folklore all the time, and how present-day events can affirm older beliefs: the tree symbolises survival, made all the more powerful by its long history as such a symbol.

Strawberries

 Sweetly fragrant in both taste and scent, strawberries are woven into happy summer memories for many people in Europe. They were reputed to be a favourite of the Norse goddess Frigg, who presided over marriages, their colour and sweetness connect them often to love and abundance. In Bavarian folk tradition, strawberries are hung in baskets on the horns of cattle as offerings to the nature spirits to request healthy calves and an abundance of milk.

English Nursery Rhyme

Curly locks! curly locks! wilt thou be mine?
Thou shalt not wash dishes, nor yet feed the swine;
But sit on a cushion and sow a fine seam,
And feed upon strawberries, sugar, and cream!

VEGETABLES IN FOLKLORE

We often think of fruit in fairy tales, but plants loosely associated with the vegetable kingdom also have magical significance: from toadstools to turnips, cabbage patches to potatoes. Jack and his beans from which a magical beanstalk grows, and through which he finds the gateway to a world of giants, and the pea that disturbs the sleep of a future princess. The pumpkin in Charles Perrault's version of "Cinderella" (1697), and the beans and lentils in the Grimm's version (1812). In this lesser-known Grimm version, Cinderella must sort through piles of lentils and peas, she is aided in this task by some pigeons.

The theme of sorting peas/beans/lentils comes up a few times in fairy tales, and is also found in the trials of Psyche, a fable that can be found in *Metamorphoses* (later named the *Golden Ass*), by Apuleius, written in the second century CE. As one of Psyche's four trials set by goddess Aphrodite, in order for her to be with her love, Cupid, Psyche must sort a heap of barley, beans, lentils and poppy seeds into separate piles, and the task seems impossible until an army of ants comes to her aid.

Beans and Peas

Strictly legumes, rather than vegetables, beans and peas have been a nutritious high-protein staple in most cultures for centuries.

Bean plants' black-spotted flowers and hollow stems caused some to think the plants connected earth and Hades, like a tiny tunnel for souls to travel or communicate.

In ancient Rome, beans were associated with the souls of the dead; they were eaten at funerals and for commemoration. Early Romans also cooked fava beans (also known as broad beans) with sage at festivals or funerals. And around the feast of All Saints and All Souls, it is still a tradition throughout Italy to eat biscuits called *fave dei morti* literally meaning "beans of the dead." Once made with fava beans, nuts are now a more popular main ingredient, and it is just the shape now that recalls the bean. One may still honour the tradition by leaving a bowl of these biscuits out overnight for the spirits.

The bean plant has similar connection in England, where souls of the dead were thought to dwell in the flowers of the bean plant: white flowers in general seem to be connected to death in lore.

The Straw, The Coal, and The Bean

A very short story from The Original Folk and Fairy Tales of the Brothers Grimm.

A piece of straw, a lump of coal and a bean are travelling together in a merry band when they come across a wide stream. They ponder how they might cross it when the straw has an idea. He lays himself over the flowing water and the coal attempts to roll over him, but burns the straw and they both fall in water and are carried off by the current. The bean laughs so hard at the misfortune of her companions, that she bursts. Luckily a tailor is able to sew her back together with thread, and this is supposedly why beans have a seam along them!

On the festive event of Twelfth Night, at revelries throughout Europe, a great cake would be served with a bean hidden somewhere within it. The person who obtained the bean was proclaimed King of the Bean, Bean King or who we know more commonly as the Lord of Misrule in England. The King of the Bean was enthroned, saluted by all and would oversee revelries and games. And perhaps, most importantly, he would make crosses with chalk on the beams and rafters of a dwelling to protect for the whole year against injury, harm, demons and witchcraft. Variations of the hidden bean in the cake are seen still in various winter celebration cakes in England, Ireland and France, though in many places the bean has become a coin, charm or ceramic figure.

The Princess and the Pea

This version is drawn from an early one by Hans Christian Anderson called "The Real Princess", which would later be renamed "The Princess and the Pea."

The extremes are interesting in this tale. The princess feels the pea through all the mattresses, suggesting she is very delicate, and sensitive, which we sometimes connect with weakness. But consider this: she makes her way through a raging storm to arrive at the castle. Then after a full night deprived of sleep, she offers an answer to appease the Old Queen and within twelve hours of arriving in the castle has bagged herself a very picky prince. So maybe she is not so weak after all...

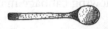

There was once a prince who wished to marry. He travelled all round the world, and met many a royal maiden, but he could not seem to find one who he considered a 'true princess.' So when he returned home he was quite out of spirits.

Now, one evening a terrible storm rolled through the kingdom; thunder and lightning crashed, and rain lashed. In the midst of it, there came a knock at the castle doors, and the guards brought a young woman through to be seen by the king and queen. She claimed to be a princess. But what a state she was in! The water trickled from her hair and clothes, and ran out of her shoes; yet she insisted she was a real princess.

"Very well," thought the Old Queen, "then we shall see." She invited this possible princess to stay until the storm passed, and had her maids take her to be bathed and clothed. While this happened, she went to what would be their guest's bedchamber and took off all the bedding. She laid a single pea upon the mattress. She then ordered twenty mattresses to be stacked upon the pea and twenty eiderdown blankets on top of those.

When night fell, the princess retired and lay upon this bed. In the morning, the Old Queen asked how she had slept. "Oh, miserably!" she said. "I scarcely closed my eyes the whole night through. I cannot think what there could have been in the bed. I lay upon something so hard that I am quite black and blue all over!"

This proved to the Old Queen that she was a real princess, since through twenty mattresses and twenty eiderdowns she had felt the pea. None but a real princess could be so delicate. So, the prince took her for his wife, for he knew that in her he had found a true princess. And the pea was preserved in the cabinet of curiosities, where it is still to be seen...

Cabbages

Native to Britain, cabbage leaves have been used in folk medicine to reduce soreness and swelling, and chewing cabbage may be prescribed for headache, cold, and flu.

On the Shetland Islands, cabbages were thrown through open doors and down chimneys on Hallow's Eve, possibly to scare off any trows[*] or to appease them, as some folklore says these creatures dwell in cabbage patches. Before churning her butter, the Shetland housewife may place a cabbage leaf and a coin under the churn, to prevent a trow from taking the profit.[7]

Cabbages are thought best planted on a new moon, perhaps in a sympathetic idea that as the moon grows to fullness, as do the plants.

And, of course, the cabbage patch is connected to birth and babies... In Victorian England babies were said to arrive via storks or from cabbage patches to avoid referring to any unseemly bodily or biological functions. And there is a saying in France, "les filles sont nées dans les roses et les garçons dans les choux" ("girls are born in the roses, and boys in the cabbages").

Lettuce

Thought to have healing and magical properties, lettuce was eaten at Roman banquets to counteract the effect of wine. The Romans also named it, derived

---

[*]   Hill creatures similar to trolls found in the folklore of the Shetland and Orkney Islands, off the northern coast of Scotland.

from the Latin word *latucca,* which refers to the vegetable's milky sap that they thought helped one have a good night's sleep. The Anglo-Saxons may well have thought the same as they called wild lettuce "sleepwort." And Culpeper in his book *The Complete Herbal* connected lettuce to the moon, so more connotations of night-time and sleep.

Seaweed

The folklore of seaweed exists in fishing villages all round the British Isles. Hanging seaweed outside your house would help predict the weather, dry seaweed means the weather will be sunny; if it's wet and flexible, rain is coming. Because it is a product of the sea and in itself salty, it could deter evil spirits in the same way as salt charms. Braids of seaweed might be hung outside the doors to prevent bad luck and drive away evil, while ships were sometimes festooned with braided seaweeds to ensure a safe voyage. In Cornwall, seaweed was sometimes called "ladies' trees," and dried small branches were hung in chimneys and around fireplaces to protect houses from fire. In spring, offerings might be made to the sea in a request for the waves to give up generous seaweed upon the shore during the spring high tides, which was used as fuel and to fertilise the fields.

Mushrooms

Fungi have some particularly delightful folklore and mushrooms and toadstools have long been connected to fairies and magic.

Mushrooms are a free, wild food that can be plentiful but, one must be mindful that many are poisonous, and in order to locate them one may well need to wander into the deep dark woods. So, one may approach mushrooms with excitement but also a healthy dose of trepidation.

You can often see the connections and superstitions applied to a foodstuff by the common, or folk names they are given, and mushrooms are particularly blessed in their names, even from just UK and European species we have: witches' butter, fairy ring champignon, witches' hats, elf cups, angel's wings, and destroying angel. Some of which can be put into a stew (fairy ring champignon), some that will kill you (destroying angel and angel's wings), and a few that will have you seeing a few fairies and other mythical creatures, in no time, as you hallucinate (witches' hats).* Some species of mushroom even glow in the dark, which adds to their magical allure. Some of the oldest recorded documentation of bioluminescence created by fungi is from ancient Greek philosopher Aristotle who named it "fox fire."

Dancing in Circles: Fairy Rings

The fairies, it's said, like to make fairy circles with the mushrooms, but should you look upon a mushroom or circle of mushrooms, they will disappear, and certainly, mushrooms and fungus circles can pop up overnight. In Holland, the circle of mushrooms was said to be where the devil rested his milk churn (that he'd possibly stolen…).

Certain mushrooms grow in circular formations, which is a naturally occurring phenomenon of underground networks of fibres that form around favourable spots in fields and forests. Folklore across Europe suggests fairy rings are the dwelling place of fairies, elves, witches, and other magical beings, tiny realms where spirits dance and play. But woe betide any human who may interrupt the fun…in some English and Celtic tales, should you enter a fairy ring, you will be compelled to dance with the fairies until you go mad or collapse.

Onions

Mars owns them, and they have gotten this quality, to draw any corruption to them, for if you peel one, and lay it upon a dunghill, you shall find it rotten in half a day, by drawing putrefaction to it.

Nicholas Culpeper, *The Complete Herbal* (1653)

Culpeper refers to a common idea, still held by many today,

---

* There are more than one kind of mushroom named witches' hats, so don't take this as an invitation to go out looking for hallucinogenic fungi.

that onions absorb germs. And if suspended in a room, onions were thought to possesses both power to attract and absorb maladies in the air, but also to drive away such evils as the Devil and witches, a power one may well see as magical. Every now and then in old buildings and pubs around England an old charm might be found consisting of an onion stuck with pins. One such discovery was made at Barley Mow in Rockwell Green, in Somerset in the early 1900s. These charms are often found in chimneys of homes – as they offer a portal into the building.

Onion skins can also be used for dying, a common use was for colouring Easter eggs yellow; the resulting eggs can be both decorative and protective.

Potatoes

A dietary mainstay in the British Isles, this root vegetable is said to be best planted on Good Friday, because the Devil has no control on this day.

Brought to Ireland and England in the 1560s by explorers who had visited South America, there was at first some reluctance to eating them as they were considered poisonous. Around the 1700s some communities of Scotland prohibited the growing of potatoes on the grounds that they are in the unholy nightshade family, and not mentioned in the Bible. (Tomatoes, also in the nightshade family, were similarly feared, but lucky for us both were accepted in time!)

Wishes might be made when the first potatoes of the year are eaten. In Shetland, the *Tattie Craa* is a potato crow made by sticking feathers into a potato, and throwing it into the air to scare away evil! A potato carried in a pocket was once a charm against rheumatism in England.

Radishes

A vegetable with peppery tasting leaves and roots, there is a superstition in Germany that wild radish, if used in a headdress, enables the wearer to detect witches. The same wreath may also protect cows and their milk.

Rapunzel the Radish

In the earliest versions of the fairy tale "Rapunzel," as told by Brothers Grimm, the couples longing for a child is mirrored in the wife's longing for rapunzel – which, at the beginning of the story is not the daughter but another name for rampion (Campanula rapunculus), an edible salad green with radish-like roots. Once widely grown in Europe, rampion's old name in German was rapunzel.

This is a strange and fascinating story about radishes, desire, and what one might do for love.

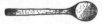

Once upon a time there lived a man and his wife who had wished dearly for a child. Finally, the woman became pregnant. At the back of their little house overlooked the garden of a sorceress skilled in growing all kinds of beautiful flowers and herbs. Nobody ever dared to enter the garden, but one day, when the wife was standing at the window and looking down into the garden, she noticed a bed of wonderful looking rapunzel. She had a great craving to eat some of it, and yet she knew that she couldn't get any. Wanting to eat only the rapunzel, she began to waste away. Her husband loved her very much so no matter the cost he was going to retrieve some rapunzel. He climbed the high wall into the garden, grabbed a handful of rapunzel, and brought the plant to his wife who ate it with great zest. However, the rapunzel tasted so very good that her craving for it became three times greater.

When he went into the garden again, he was terrified to come face-to-face with the sorceress, who scolded him for daring to come into the garden and steal her rapunzel. He explained that his wife was pregnant and that it had become too dangerous to deny her this food she so wanted. "All right," the sorceress said. "I shall permit you to take as much rapunzel as you like. But only if you give me the child that your wife is carrying." In his fear the man agreed to everything.

When his wife gave birth, the sorceress appeared at once. She took the baby away and locked her in a high tower. She named the baby girl Rapunzel. As the baby girl grew, so did her locks of fine, strong, golden hair.

And soon, whenever the sorceress wanted to enter the tower, she would stand below and call out, "Rapunzel, Rapunzel, let down your hair." And Rapunzel let down her golden braids so that the sorceress could climb up.

One day a young prince was riding through the forest and came upon the tower. He looked up and saw beautiful Rapunzel at the window. He went into the forest every day until one time he saw the sorceress, who called out, "Rapunzel, Rapunzel, let down your hair." He took careful note of the words he had to say.

The next day, he went to the tower and called out, "Rapunzel, Rapunzel, let down your hair." Rapunzel let her hair drop, and up he climbed.

At first Rapunzel was wary. But soon the young prince pleased her so much that she agreed to see him every day. They had a merry time and enjoyed each other's company. The sorceress didn't become aware of this until, one day, Rapunzel said to her, "Why are my clothes becoming too tight? They don't fit around my belly anymore."

The sorceress became furious, she grabbed Rapunzel's beautiful hair and *snip, snap,* cut it off. She banished Rapunzel to a desolate land, where she gave birth to twins. On the same day that the sorceress had banished Rapunzel, the prince came by and called out, "Rapunzel, Rapunzel, let down your hair."

But this time it was the sorceress who let the cut braids down. When the prince climbed up into the tower, there was no Rapunzel, only an angry sorceress who cried, "You villain! Rapunzel is lost to you forever!"

In his despair the prince threw himself from the tower. He escaped with his life, but he lost sight in both eyes. He wandered the forest, eating nothing but grass and roots, and did nothing but weep. Some years later, he made his way to the desolate land where Rapunzel was leading a wretched existence with her children. When he heard her voice, he recognized it, and she embraced him. Two of her tears fell upon his eyes, and he could see once more.

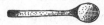

In later versions of the tale it was confirmed that they did live happily ever after, which is comforting after this pretty traumatic series of incidents.

Another Woman in a Tower...

This is a very short version of the story of Princess Mayblossom (Princesse Printaniére), from Fairy Tales (Les Contes des Fées) *by Marie-Catherine d'Aulnoy (1697) as translated by Annie Macdonell and Miss Lee (1892).*

I was delighted to find this story as not only does it have some lovely food imagery but also features a princess who is cursed by circumstance beyond her control, makes some unwise choices, but ultimately seizes her skills and power to find her own 'happy ever after.' Also, the fact that hunger and thirst act as catalyst — as well as some wise plants — to reveal, her love's true nature.

A king and queen named their newly born daughter Mayblossom, for she was as bright as the spring and as beautiful as lilies and roses. But they despaired when the new-born princess was cursed by a malevolent fairy to be miserable her first twenty years of life. A fairy godmother was brought in to help, and she did what she could to remedy the curse by assuring that Princess Mayblossom's life would be long and happy after those first twenty years and advised that the princess be kept in a tower to minimize the harm up to her twentieth year.

Now, leading up to her twentieth birthday many ambassadors to kings visited the tower to propose matches for the princess who would soon be free to wed. One fateful day, Princess Mayblossom, peeking through a hole in the tower wall, beheld one such ambassador and she instantly fell in love with him and called out to him. With his help, she escaped the tower and they ran away, taking with them the king's dagger and the queen's headdress. They fled to a nearby desert island.

Once upon this island, the ambassador began to complain of hunger and thirst, and when the princess could find nothing for him, he suddenly found himself falling very quickly, out of love.

Nevertheless, she kept looking through the island for food, and eventually came across a beautiful red rose. The flower offered her some sparkling sweet honeycomb but warned her not to show the ambassador.

However, still seeking to please him, she did, and he snatched up the golden honeycomb and ate it all, leaving nothing for her.

The next day, the princess found an old oak tree that offered her a pitcher of creamy milk but warned her not to show the ambassador. Once again she did, and once again he snatched it up and drank it all.

The princess began to despair in her rash choice to elope. But, that evening with gentle wings a nightingale arrived to her and offered her sugarplums and delicious little fruit tarts. This time, she was quiet and ate them, with great joy, herself.

When the ambassador discovered she had eaten without him, he threatened her. But being wise to magic she took up the queen's headdress, that she had brought with her, and placed it on her head. Within her mother's headdress was an enchanted stone that made her invisible. The hungry and furious ambassador tried to kill her and eat her, but she killed him first with the help of the king's dagger.

By now men had been sent to seek out the princess, and she alone was brought back to the kingdom. Upon her twentieth birthday she sought and found herself a fine prince and she lived with him, happily ever after.

NUTS

Nuts were, and are, a free food source if they can be found in the wild, which made them hugely valuable to folks during 'need years' and through long winter months. To "go a' nutting" was an enjoyable pastime around September for rural communities in many European countries. A precious source of fats, the nut's value is often reflected in their role in folk and fairy tales where nut shells often contain 'treasure' of some kind.

Christmas Nut Cracking

The Nutcracker is a decorative soldier figure with very strong jaws, made in Germany and now famous the world over at Christmastime. This fame is thanks not only the designer who created the wooden nutcracker figure but also the creatives who were inspired to weave story around the figures. German author E.T.A. Hoffmann wrote "The Nutcracker and the Mouse King" in 1816, which Tchaikovsky would turn into a ballet in 1892. It is still a Christmas classic, shown widely every winter, and has become part of many families' treasured Christmas customs.

Jacob Grimm wrote about Nutcrackers briefly in *Deutsche Mythologie* in 1835.

> *Wooden Nutcrackers and other mere playthings are cut in the shape of a dwarf or idol; yet the practice may have had to do with an old heathen worship of small lares, to whom a place was assigned in the innermost part of the dwelling.*

He likened the wooden Nutcrackers to protective figures, like home sprites to protect homes and ward off evil spirits. Nutcrackers were, and still are, gifted at Christmas to bring good luck to the family and home, as well as a guardian over the treasured ritual of cracking nuts, drinking and gathering round the fire with friends and family. This is a great example of how Nutcrackers have, been subject and inspiration for (relatively) new folklore and superstitions based around them – drawn from both their practical use, historical comparisons to older customs and stories they have inspired.

Hazelnuts

The crunchy, sweet hazelnut is even sweeter once roasted, and a modern favourite for adding to chocolate treats. Magical hazel trees in Celtic lore, were a connection to the otherworld and grew over sacred pools. Their nuts fell into the water and drifting downstream, were eaten by a salmon that would become the Salmon of Knowledge in Irish legends. Anyone who ate these hazelnuts, or the salmon would gain wisdom and poetic skill. In Norse mythology, the hazel tree was known as a tree of knowledge and to Romans, as Culpeper notes in his Herbal, was held sacred to Mercury, who personified intelligence.

Walnuts

Earthy walnut flesh can taste a little bitter, but in fairy tales, walnuts are often mentioned as dispensers of gifts. Within them, there is often something beautiful, precious, or nourishing. A nutritionist would well know walnuts contain fatty acids that support brain function; supporting a folk belief that foods that look like a body part also support that area, and walnuts do look like little brains!

In "The Iron Stove" (Brothers Grimm), a princess receives three nuts as a gift, which are sometimes identified as walnuts. Within each nut, a magnificent dress magically appears: the colours of the stars, moon and sun in turn. In "The Children of the Two Kings" also by the Brothers Grimm, walnut shells also hold clothing inside. And a Hungarian fairy tale called "The Little Walnut" sees the nut furnish a poor man with all the riches he desires. There are many versions of the tale of walnuts holding abundance in beautiful dresses throughout Europe and in a Tuscan version, it's a tiny dog with golden collar decorated with tinkling bells that leaps from the nut.

The walnut has mainly positive connotations but the walnut tree less so. Because the canopy of the black walnut tree is so dense, little can grow underneath the shadow it casts and if planted in an orchard a walnut tree can kill neighbouring apple trees (The black walnut tree secretes a chemical from its roots into the soil that is toxic to other plants).

This shadowy silhouette and unneighbourly conduct meant that the ancient Romans considered the walnut tree to be a bit sinister. Which in turn brought up imagery of the Underworld and Persephone and her infernal spirit friends, witches included. The tree gathered a reputation as a favourite haunt of witches and an ill-omen throughout Italy for many centuries after the time of the Roman Empire.

The Witches' Walnut Tree

The most infamous walnut tree may well be the Walnut Tree of Benevento, Italy, around which, witches were said to dance. The history and legend of the witches of Benevento is now folklore of the region.[8] And the popular belief of the connection of witches and walnut trees ran from superstition into the real-life witch hunts (not the first or last time folklore would influence real-life witch trials).

Though the tree is no longer standing, texts have referred to the tree in essays and poems for centuries. And some of those say it stood on the banks of the Sabato River, and was site to magical and pagan practices, and ancient goddess cults to Diana, Artemis, Hecate and Isis.

The legends developed to include witches in flight, gathering and dancing under the great walnut tree as a hub for Italian witches' Sabbats, similar to the Brocken Mountain in Germany and Blakulla island in Sweden (more on these later). And the witch fable has been wholeheartedly embraced by the local distillers of Strega (witch) liqueur, created in 1833 and now distributed worldwide. (The witches are still dancing around their walnut tree on the bottle's label.)

Almonds

Like many nuts, almonds have long been a symbol of fertility and prosperity. In ancient Greece and Rome, creamy, sweet almonds dipped in honey were given to newlyweds, and to celebrate births. And when sugar became more readily available, the almonds were coated with a hard sugar shell. Still today sugar-coated almonds are often given to guests at weddings. In Italy each guest is given five almonds to represent five wishes: health, wealth, happiness, fertility, and longevity for the newlyweds.

Almonds for Scented Goddesses

Almonds were valuable not just as food, but as perfume. In an archaeological dig in 2003 on the island of Cyprus, the oldest perfumery found to date was unearthed by archaeologist Dr. Maria Rosaria Belgiorno. Perfume bottles, amphorae and stills were found preserved under the collapsed walls, along with finished perfumes, recipes and remains of their ingredients: laurel, lavender, rosemary, anise, pine, coriander, bergamot, and parsley, and almonds. Sweet almond oil could be used as a base and bitter almond was used to provide sweet scent.

Later Dr. Belgiorno and her team helped recreate some of the perfumes from remains found in little alabaster phials: they sit alongside the perfumery artifacts in the Capitolini Museum in Rome. They named them after the ancient Greek goddesses: Artemis, Hera, Athena and Aphrodite.

Artemis contained olive oil, almonds, myrtle, parsley and turpentine. *Hera*: olive oil, rosemary, green anise and lavender. *Athena*: olive oil, laurel, coriander and turpentine. *Aphrodite*: olive oil, pine, turpentine and bergamot.

Gilda and the Almond Blossoms
– a Portuguese folk tale*

Once upon a time the Algarve was ruled by a young Moorish prince. He fell in love with Gilda, a princess from Norway, daughter of a great lord from the North. Their marriage was celebrated in grand style, and the newlyweds were both very joyful. However, in time, the beautiful princess grew sad, a little more each day, like a sickness that crept over her and made her weep. The prince, worried for his love, consulted magicians and wise men, but none could find a cure for her sadness…

One day an old Nordic man appeared with an answer for the young prince. He said that Gilda was longing for the white snow-covered fields of her Norwegian homeland. The prince could not bring the Nordic snow to Portugal, but he devised a plan to do the next best thing. He ordered that thousands of almond trees be planted in front of the palace, lining the gardens, outside the windows, down the hills and far into the countryside. And when they came into blossom, the prince brought Gilda to the windows of the palace to see how they covered the land with white petals that glistened in the sun like freshly fallen snow. Gilda gasped and felt her heart lift at the beauty of this sight. She never felt homesick again, and she and her prince lived happily ever after.

And since that spring so long ago, the Algarve relives each year the magic of the almond blossom heralding the arrival of spring, bathing the land in a dazzling snow.

---

* This version is from the Portuguese tourism website at visitalgarve.pt where the beautiful cultural stories of their folklore are woven amongst timeless enticements for tourists like beaches, sunshine and food.

HERBS AND SEASONINGS

Throughout the world, spices and herbs are frequently used in cooking for flavour and preservation, but also for nourishment and healing, underlining the fact that throughout cultures and history food was medicine, and medicine was food.

Herbal medicine and the use of herbs in cooking have been practised since the first ancient civilisations. Many of the herbs we use today have been known for thousands of years, just as effective now as they were then. Turmeric, which is now widely lauded for its anti-inflammatory properties, and pretty trendy with its reincarnation in turmeric lattes at Starbucks and juice bars, has been used in Ayurvedic medicine for thousands of years. Similarly, fennel was used in relieving digestive problems in the Middle Ages, and we still use it today to soothe and calm, especially in tea blends, by the likes of big tea companies such as Pukka and Twinings.

Modern scholars and historians may well think that in the past, people knew that plant remedies worked, but not why; I think they did understand, just perhaps in different ways to how we quantify these things now.

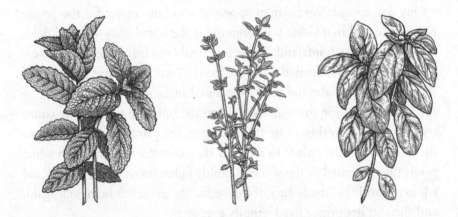

You might say that herbs exist in a space between science and wonder, medicine and magic, spell craft and holistic wellbeing. We can create our own relationships with herbs and receive just a little bit of their magic. Herbs and spices are potent and powerful, and while you don't have to connect to this rich history and power when using herbs in order for them to work, wouldn't it be wonderful to, every now and then, peek inside this treasure trove of ancient wisdom and magic and release it into your body and the modern world!

Parsley

A mild flavoured herb that is high in nutrients. Some say only a witch can grow parsley, and certainly other malevolent beings seem to have varying influence on this herb. Its seeds are one of the slowest to germinate, and so the story arose that the seeds go to the Devil and back again nine times before the plant grows. But if you wanted to grow it fast, it should be planted on a Good Friday, supposedly a day that the Devil has no power.

Ancient Greeks and Romans both connected parsley to death in some way, but it was also thought sacred – so wreaths might be used for both mourning and celebration. It is also useful to eat after a meal for digestion and fresher breath.

Angelica

The beautifully named angelica (*Angelica archangelica*) is a perennial herb commonly known as wild celery. It is used as a traditional medicine in Europe and Russia, where it grows wild. The roots of angelica are used to make herbal medicines to treat a wide range of conditions ranging from heartburn, digestive problems, and insomnia. Today, as well as medicine, the herb is used in cooking; stems can be used in salads and candied as sweets and leaves can go into soups and stews. It is also used for flavouring for alcoholic beverages such as gin and Bénédictine.

As you might expect from a plant named for the angels, it was used to protect from witches, elves, evils, and enchantments. According to folklore, angelica is named after an angel that, appearing before a monk in plague-ridden Europe, showed him to the angelica plant as a cure. Or because it flowers on St. Michael's Day[*] – as noted below...

> *The umbelliferous plant, it has been supposed, has been named Angelica archangelica, from its being in blossom on the 8th of May, old style, the Archangel St. Michael's Day. Flowering on the fête day of such a powerful angel, the plant was supposed to be particularly useful as a preservative of men and women from evil spirits and witches, and of cattle from elfshot...*

---

[*]   In the Roman Catholic Church calendar there is a feast to celebrate the event of the Apparition of St. Michael the Archangel on May 8, as well as Michaelmas in September.

its roots, worn suspended round the neck, would guard the wearer against the baneful power of witches and enchantments; and Gerard tells us that a piece of the root held in the mouth, or chewed, will drive away pestilential air, and that the plant, besides being a singular remedy against poisons, the plague, and pestilent diseases in general, cures the biting of mad dogs and all other venomous beasts.

Richard Folkard, *Plant Lore, Legends, and Lyrics* (1884)

Rosemary

Rosemary (from *ros marinus* meaning "dew of the sea") is a waxy needle-leafed aromatic herb that has been used in Europe, Asia and the Americas as a herbal medicine for centuries, dating back to the ancient Egyptians. In the fourteenth century, the herb was burned in houses to keep the Black Death from entering. Rosemary is still used as an ingredient for incense today and used to cleanse sacred spaces. It's possible that the Saxons found rosemary growing all over England because of its introduction by the Romans.

Rosemary Reflections

The ancient Greeks believed rosemary helped the memory and wore garlands of it around their heads when taking exams. It was associated with Mnemosyne, the goddess of memory, who was thought to have given humans their capacity for remembrance. As an act of mercy to ease their suffering in the afterlife, she would make them drink from Lethe, the Underworld river of forgetfulness. This folklore around memory and death has continued in England, where rosemary has been used for remembrance in funerary arrangements for centuries, as noted in Shakespeare's Hamlet where Ophelia, gathering flowers and herbs says, "rosemary, that's for remembrance".

Lucy H. Pearce, *She of the Sea* (2021)

Garlic

Pungent and full-flavoured, the ancient Egyptians, Greeks, and Romans all used garlic for medicinal, spiritual, healing and protection purposes. Today, we understand garlic to be destructive to various viruses and bacteria and an antibiotic oil called allicin found in garlic can boost the immune system. Sulfuric compounds in garlic also make it an effective repellent of some insects and animals.

The renowned Greek physician and philosopher in the Roman Empire, Galen, wrote of garlic as a cure-all, along with Hippocrates, who suggested garlic could be used for healing everything from cuts and digestive issues to cancer and leprosy. Greek midwives might hang garlic in birthing rooms to safeguard newborns against malevolent spirits.[9] This ancient custom would become commonplace in most European homes for protection and many of us still hang braids of garlic in our kitchens, sometimes just for decoration, but extra warding against evil never hurts!

So, it's the powers of protection which garlic holds that may have caused it to be connected to repelling pretty much any malevolent spirits conjured by history, superstition, and folklore, protecting people and homes. Over time, garlic became a warding item for many creatures including vampires, devils, demons, evil spirits...and witches according to Emily Gerard, a Scottish nineteenth-century author best-known for her collections of Transylvanian folklore (her work is credited with inspiring Bram Stoker to write *Dracula* in 1897!). "In bringing in the corn a few heads of garlic bound up in the first sheaf will keep off witches."[10]

Vampiric Sidenote

Vampiric spirits, demons, and the notion of vampirism have been recorded in most ancient cultures: night-roaming spirits who feast on the blood, energy, and flesh of mortals. Vampires, like witches, have been drawn through history in various guises and have roots in folklore, demonology, and images from mythology. In Greco-Roman mythology we find the Lamia and Strix, monstrous female demons who preyed on young children and adults in their beds at night, sucking their blood. And Empusa, daughter of goddess Hecate, was feared to first seduce and then feast on the flesh of young men in their bedchambers. In Europe around the mid-1700s when both fear and fascination of demons, devils and witches was high, pre-existing folk beliefs and superstitions were built upon to create new devils especially in poetry and later in fictional tales, to bring the vampires as we know them today, to life (or not, as the case may be!).

Honey

For thousands of years, honey has sweetened our food as well as being the chief ingredient in early intoxicating beverages like mead and honey wine. Honey was used as an ancient preservative and all the way up to World War II to clean wounds, making use of its antimicrobial benefits.

Today we are more aware than ever of the value of bees for our ecosystem. In folklore bees represent abundance, both of the land and environment and in the quantities of sweet honey they produce. Bees are little alchemists, collecting the nectar of the land and turning it into gold that is both nourishing and delicious, so delicious, in fact, to earn it a place as a sacred food. Honey was used in offerings and libations of the ancient Greeks, who considered it the "nectar of the gods." In Greek myth, when Zeus was in his infancy, he was stowed away in a cavern that was home to hives of sacred bees. There he was fed on goat's milk and honey. The ancient Greeks also believed that in addition to a coin for payment to the ferryman of the River Styx, the dead should also bring a honey cake: a pacifying gift for Cerberus, the three-headed guard dog of the Underworld. The goddess Psyche placates the dog in this way as part of her four trials set by Aphrodite.

In Germany, honey might be given as a housewarming or wedding gift to sweeten the marriage. And, as well as the honeymoon, widely thought to refer to the 'sweetest' time of marriage, there are also various customs including Celtic and Anglo-Saxon, where couples drink mead, or honey-wine during the marriage ceremony for fertility and abundance.

Celtic mythology held that bees were the link between our world and the spirit world, considered either messengers of the gods, or embodiments of the gods themselves. It was wise to notify the bees of a death in the family, so that they could share in the mourning or perhaps pass on messages of love to those who had passed. The practice of 'telling the bees' has been recorded across Europe and the rural United States for centuries. If it is the bee's keeper, often the head of the household that has died, as well as words, food was offered to the bees, biscuits might be soaked in wine and left out for the bees in offering so that they may have a tiny funerary feast of their own for their master.

Salt

If an old woman is suspected of being a witch, it is the custom to throw a hand-ful of salt after her, when, if she really is a witch, she will look round. When anyone who is thought to be a witch will enter a house, it is merely necessary to place a broom inverted in the doorway: if she is a witch, she cannot enter. [*]

Northern Mythology: Popular Traditions and Superstitions of Scandinavia, North Germany, and the Netherlands, compiled by Benjamin Thorpe

Salt features in numerous fairy tales and superstitions around the world. A high-value commodity, spilling it was always considered bad luck.

Most have heard the story of the word salary, which comes from the word *sal*, Roman soldiers were paid in salt and this is thought to be the origin of the phrase to be "worth one's salt". As well as a valued seasoning, salt was a preserver of food (and the dead), so most superstitions see salt as protective or cleansing in some way. Throwing a pinch of salt over your left shoulder, where the Devil was thought to sit, would blind him. You would be protected from harm, ill omens and bad luck. One might throw salt on the floor of a new house for protection or throw it into the hearth fire. Notice how intention plays a pivotal role: salt thrown with purpose is protective, spilt carelessly is bad luck.

In England, salt may protect one from witches and reverse bad spells (it's always fascinating how the practices of witches and guarding against them are often one and the same). Sprinkling salt on the doorstep of your home after

---

[*]   These are interesting reflections on both salt and broomsticks, which in other lore are pretty appealing to the witch!

an unwanted visitor had left would stop them from returning. Today, salt is still used in some pagan and witchcraft practices to create a circle of protection. It is popular in modern-day witchcraft practice on altars and in baths as a cleanser, both spiritual and physical. Salt is essential to health, but too much can kill you, and we see that dual potential again of witches and healing potions: both can heal *and* harm.

There are a *lot* of religions and countries that believe in using salt to cleanse and ward off evil spirits.

☾ Irish folk remedies include the use of salt and a recitation of the Lord's Prayer to cure those who might have been "fairy-struck."

☾ In Da Vinci's renowned artwork "The Last Supper," we can see, if we look carefully, Judas has spilled a bottle of salt on the table! Possibly a little joke in the painting about Judas being up to no good and the bad fortune he will invite into the group.

☾ If someone spills salt, it can mean a quarrel is on the way. If you do spill salt, throw it over your left shoulder. Your left ear being the one that the Devil whispers into, so throwing salt over your left shoulder should send him on his way!

☾ In parts of northern England and Scotland it can be bad luck to lend salt to others: the person borrowing it can use it as a magical link to curse you.

☾ In Norse and Danish fairy tales the sea is salty because of a magic coffee mill, running out of control: it begins grinding salt, and never stops. In similar tales and poems from Norway, Iceland and Orkney it is two giant-esses Fenyeh and Menyeh who grind a giant quernstone. When invaders appeared on their land, a foreign king took the giantesses and the quern on his ship and asked them to grind salt. They do, but in something of a rebellion, continue until the ship sinks under the weight of it all, and the giantesses still grind the salt at the bottom of the sea.

I Love You More Than Salt

Versions of this story can be found throughout Europe, the central theme being not to dismiss the value of something as everyday as salt.

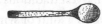

There was once an old king who asked his daughters how much they loved him. He was delighted to hear his first daughter say, "I love you more than gold and silver," and equally when the second daughter said, "I love you more than diamonds and rubies and pearls."

But when his third and youngest daughter answered, "I love you more than salt," the king was furious for comparing her love to something so common and banished her from his kingdom. In her exile, the princess met a kindly old crone who took her in and taught her how to weave and cook in her little cottage. The princess was a good worker and didn't complain, but her heart ached for her father and that he had misunderstood her love so completely.

Meanwhile, that common salt which the king had derided, well, it had vanished from the realm! Every last grain. And strange chaos descended on the kingdom. The king and his people became weak and sickly without salt; all food had lost its flavour. The king's favourites – oatmeal, pies, roast meats – none of them pleased him now. Nothing tasted the same.

Many months later, the old crone told the girl it was time for her to return to her family and handed her a small bag of salt.

The crone, you see, had hidden all the salt in the kingdom and far beyond, to teach the old king a lesson. And when the princess returned to the castle, the guards stopped her at the gate, but she pulled out her bag of salt and handed it to them. They rejoiced. The king welcomed her home and threw a great feast in her honour and apologised for his foolishness. From that day on, the kingdom never suffered from a lack of love...or salt.

BREAD AND WHEAT

Farming communities all over the world have superstitions and rituals for ensuring, as best they can, a successful harvest. Once, the whole community of a village would have been involved in harvesting the grain: men reaping, women and children gathering and tying into sheaves. The fortunes of the communities relied on it, and harvest traditions and rituals were created to encourage its success in a kind of sympathetic folk magic. Cornish farmers when winnowing wheat would whistle to the wind spirits for their help separating the grains from the chaff when tossing in the air. The work of separating grains is a challenge that appears in a fair few fairy tales. In Grimm's fairy tales, such tasks are set with millet seeds, poppy seeds, peas and as I have said in "Cinderella," she must pick peas and lentils out of ashes before she is allowed to go to the ball.

From wheat, rye, barley, and oats came many staples of the historic diet: bread, beer, oatcakes, porridge…it is no wonder, then, that these foodstuffs feature so frequently in the folklore of so many cultures.

Bread Tales in Eastern Europe

Slavic tales offer many versions of how people learned to bake bread. Depending on the storyteller, bread was gifted by dragons, the gods, or demons. And like in many cultures, holiday celebrations usually involved the consumption of bread, baking as a gift to others, or as an offering to deities or ancestors. Breadcrumbs might be cast onto graves for the birds, as they represented ancestral souls.

Russian healers used different parts of bread in healing various ailments. The bread crust, because it touched the hot metal of the bread pan, was associated with the element of fire, while the rest of it represents the life-giving role of the earth. The dough, kneaded by hand, was considered a powerfully charged magical object, as the woman who kneaded it added her own thoughts and wishes into the dough. Cooks would recite incantations and prayers when kneading dough for a ritual bread, such as ring-shaped ritual breads for weddings and Christmas, and Spring Equinox buns called "larks" (bread shaped as little birds to invite in the spring season).

Bread and Gold – a Slavic tale

A wise sorceress asked two men, "What is more precious: bread or gold?"

"Gold is more precious than bread," says one man.

"Bread is more precious than gold," says the other, who is a farmer.

The sorceress gives each one the thing they considered more precious: piles of shining gold to the first man and piles of all kinds of bread to the farmer, and then leaves them both locked up separate from each other for several days.

When she checks on the first man, he is dead, but the farmer is not only still alive but completely content. Gold is only valuable when you're surrounded by other people that could trade you bread for that gold. When you just have bread on your table you need nothing more.

In folk tradition, baking bread was often compared to the birth of a human being (seen in the common saying, "a bun in the oven," to refer to pregnancy). In a skill once practised widely throughout Eastern Europe, a healer or midwife could 're-bake' a prematurely born and sickly baby. For this, she would wrap the baby up and place it in a warm oven. After some time and careful observance, the baby was removed from the oven, born again, in a sense. The rite is intended to heal by using gentle warmth (rural farms still use this custom in the UK to revive lambs, and we use incubators in hospitals for the same purpose). But to someone who doesn't understand what's happening, it might look horrifying, and it is an image that has been hijacked and woven into scary fairy tales we most closely associate with Baba Yaga and the witch of the gingerbread house putting children into ovens.

Bad Bread Magic

The witch trials of Salem in colonial Massachusetts occurred through 1692 and 1693 and have gone down in history as one of the most extreme purges in such a small area. They saw two hundred people accused of witchcraft: nineteen of whom were executed by hanging, seven or so more died in jail, including an infant baby born to one of the accused witches, and one man was crushed to death.

There has been ongoing study and fascination into what happened in Salem. In 1976 Dr. Linnda Caporael suggested that the brief and intense illnesses suffered by so many of the townspeople in Salem during the infamous witch trials were not bewitchment but rather ergotism, a disease contracted from rye bread and the ergot fungus.[11] (Ergotism is also called Saint Anthony's Fire, St. Anthony being the patron saint of the poor, sick, and all things lost.) Ergotism can form in rye after a harsh winter and a damp spring – conditions that historians claim were present in 1691 and therefore affected the rye harvest that was eaten for the following year. Ergot fungus contains ergotamine and lysergic acid (which is useful to know because the drug LSD is synthesised from lysergic acid). Ergotism can cause severe convulsions, muscle spasms, delusions, and hallucinations. These symptoms were shown in a group of young girls in Salem, which the village doctor attributed to a known evil: witchcraft.

This is just one theory (and not a popular one with some academics), and certainly, other factors were involved. Like all witch hunts, no single variable was to blame. Townsfolk fell victim to suggestibility, fear, prejudice, religious indoctrination, social and political unrest, and thus the trials commenced, with accusations of witchcraft causing havoc. But this is an interesting consideration, and a reminder of the many ways food can play a part in events, how powerful it can be and maybe that nothing is ever quite as it seems… (Oh, and don't eat mouldy bread, that's always sound advice!)

Pancakes

Pancakes – a delicious and simple-to-make treat – are a common occurrence in folklore and fairy tale. Pancakes have existed, in various forms, for a very long time and archaeologists have found evidence of pancakes from back in the Stone Age, made from wheat as well as millet and barley. These would have been cooked over hot stones, placed on a fire. In the Middle Ages, pancakes became particularly associated with Shrove Tuesday.

In England, in the village of Toddington, Bedfordshire on Shrove Tuesday (also known as Pancake Day), in a tradition that is said to date back at least 150 years, after hearing the Parish Church "pancake bell" ring, children would run up Conger Hill and press their ears to the ground to listen for the sizzling sound of a witch frying her pancakes. Conger Hill is an ancient fortification thought to date back to the Bronze Age, so it is not impossible that pancakes were made in ancient times in and around Conger Hill. But whether it's witches making them is still up for debate.

A Pancake Fairy Tale

This is drawn from a story called "A Witch Burnt," from the Netherlands. An earlier version of this story can be found in Northern Mythology *by Benjamin Thorpe (1852).*

There is a wealth of folklore about witches and butter, and its value is apparent in many folktales of household spirits, who favour offerings of porridge with butter. In Ireland, particularly, the fear of butter bewitchment coincided with particular festivals, so I will save more butter stories for Section Four.

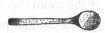

They say that the castle of Erendegen is so haunted that the ghosts bump into each other as they wisp through the walls like travelling clouds. They get tangled up sometimes and have to whirl and twist to detach themselves. Promises of gold and foolhardy bets were often made in the alehouses of Erendegen, as the villagers tried to persuade friends and passers-by to stay a night in the castle. But they never succeeded. Too cold and dark and eerie was the place, and too great their fear.

One day a man who went by the name Bold Jan stood on a table in the alehouse and boasted that he could stay any length of time at the castle, as long as he had everything he needed for frying pancakes. The villagers laughed. But they were intrigued – what would become of this strange man? Surely his adventure would make for a good tale to brighten dark evenings. And so, they gathered: a heavy pan, rich creamy butter wrapped in brown paper, hens' eggs and fine flour from the miller – all the while laughing. The village children spread flour on their faces and loomed towards their friends howling as they imagined the menacing ghosts.

Soon, the ingredients were all ready, and the crowd quietened. Dusk was falling, and Jan gathered his foods and took the short walk to the castle. The villagers waved him off and returned to their homes.

Alone at last, Jan ascended the stone steps which were grimy with age and moss. He walked through the splintered old door and into the castle. His shoes kicked up dust, and crumbled plaster crunched under his feet in a vast hallway. He could smell the damp and dirt, and some distant smells of memories long forgotten. The light was low, not helped by the grimy windows. He let his hands slide over well-worn bannisters as he made his way up the creaking stairs.

He found a grand room with a big stone fireplace and built a fire from the sticks he had gathered from the castle grounds. Soon he had a golden fire crackling in the fireplace, casting dancing light and a wave of heat through the room. He pulled a wooden chair close to the flame, and brought out his cooking utensils. He whisked up his batter and began to fry a sweet-smelling pancake on the fire.

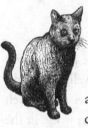

The door of the room creaked gently open. It was not a ghost but a black cat that prowled into the room, and, as cats are wont to do, she came to warm herself by the flames. "What are you doing?" she asked.

"I am frying pancakes, my little friend," said Jan. This answer seemed to be the one that the cat was seeking because as soon as the words came out of his mouth seven more cats entered the room.

This slinking clan of felines once again asked Jan what he was doing, and Jan, once again answered, "I am frying pancakes."

Again, this answer seemed favourable to the cats who, taking each other's paws, began to dance round and round in a swirling dance.

What's wrong with that? you may ask, but Jan had another plan that perhaps they would not like so much. As they danced in the firelight amongst smells of smoke and sweet pancakes, Jan filled the pan with all of the blocks of butter. The butter melted and bubbled, turning golden scalding hot. Jan threw the butter over the cats, and in one instant, they all vanished. The melted butter quickly solidified upon the floor, in pale creamy pools.

The following day, Jan was standing on a table again, this time in the village square. It was a beautiful bright autumnal day, rich blue sky above and golden leaves underfoot. The villagers emerged from their homes to hear Jan announce that the castle would be no more haunted.

With the crowd looking on at the show, the shoemaker's wife moved very slowly, she had a long fresh burn along her arm. She was in pain but allowed herself a chuckle as Jan continued the speech of his bravery, adding evermore ghosts to his story of his night in the castle. She cast a look over to the baker's wife and raised her eyebrows with an almost imperceptible smile. The baker's wife nodded and took a bite out of the day's special: a rolled pancake filled with fine buttercream. They were not done. And some soft butter on those burns would soothe them nicely.[*]

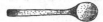

This story follows a popular folklore theme of a witch being harmed in animal form that then follows into her human form, and similar versions of this kind of tale can be found in Ireland, Wales, Scotland and England. In these stories, a witch would often be portrayed as a cat or a hare, shot by a hunter, and a woman would then appear to have the same injury. I suppose what has been 'achieved' is that a witch has been identified, but these stories reflect a rather casual attitude and acceptance of violence against both animals and women.

---

[*] The idea of putting butter on burns is something many English people remember from a time when it was also thought prudent to put a steak on a black eye and mustard could cure a cold. These folk cures are often known as "old wives tales", not necessarily false but from stories so old no one can remember the origin! Butter for burns features in *Bald's Leechbook* (c. 900), "For sunburn boil in butter tender ivy twigs, smear therewith." So it's not without provenance. I mention it in the story as a nod to that superstition, but I want to stress that the best way to cool skin after receiving a burn is with cool water!

Milk, Cream, Butter and Cheese

That story of pancakes moves us neatly on to dairy products. Milk, cheese, butter and cream were mainstays of country life, where many families would have their own cow, sheep or goat. Milk was of huge importance to our early ancestors' diet for nourishment, and high-calorie delights such as butter and cheese, would have been vital in surviving a long winter.

Many cultures revere the cow and her milk as a symbol of nurturing. In Irish mythology, the Milky Way was *Bealach na Bó Finne* – Way of the White Cow. This glowing band of stars arching across the night sky would have been more visible on dark winter nights. In Greek mythology, the Milky Way was formed after a deceptive deity (in some tellings it's the god Hermes, in others it's Athena) suckled the infant Heracles at the breast of Hera, the queen of the gods, while she was asleep, so that he would obtain divine powers. When Hera awoke, she tore Heracles away from her breast with such speed that her breast milk was scattered across the heavens. And the word galaxy is derived from the Greek *galaxias*, literally "milky," a reference to the Milky Way, but now a word we use for all star systems.

> *The Lancashire peasant, in some districts, still believes the "Milky Way" to be the path by which departed souls enter Heaven… The Germans entertain a similar belief in the "Milky Way" being the spirit path to heaven. In Friesland its name is kaupat, or cowpath.*

Charles Hardwick, *Traditions, Superstitions and Folk-lore* (1872)

St. Brigid and the Celtic goddess Brigid are both closely linked to cows and milk. In Ireland the first milk of the year gathered from the ewes might be offered to Brigid by pouring it upon the earth or made into special cheeses, bread and cakes and featured in milk dishes and drinks for the feast.

Brigid was, the legend goes, fed as a child on the milk of white faery cows and as a deity connected to fertility, she provides milk for villages that honour her, and none go hungry. The *Bonnach Bride* (Irish) or Bannock of Bride (Scottish) is an oatcake left out on the Eve of Imbolc (January 31st/ February 1st) as an offering to Brigid to hopefully gain her blessings of fertility, prosperity, and good health. Bannocks were also offered to the fields to honour the land. Anglo-Saxons would also offer bread and milk as a gift to the fields: goddesses of the grain have long been honoured in such ways.

Milk Witches

Milk's value can be seen in fear of its loss, especially on festival days, when more otherworldly beings may be abound, and malevolent witches were blamed for meddling with milk and cheese. Spoiling milk was one of the most common curses associated with witches in early modern Europe. There are also tales through the British Isles and beyond into Europe of witches stealing milk through many nefarious means, including turning themselves into hares to suckle milk directly from the cows, skimming the morning dew of farmers' fields, and in this way magically "skimming" milk from their stores.

The fairy folk, particularly, if not appeased with food offerings may also cause milk mischief: causing milk to dry up, spoiling cream or cursing the butter churn. As defence for such attacks, housewives might wrap rowan or mountain ash around their butter churns and milk pails to prevent their contents from being stolen by the fairies. This same technique was used for warding against witches. In parts of Scotland and Europe, salt sprinkled around a butter churn was believed to keep witches from souring the butter or harming the cow that produced the cream.

DRINKS

Coffee

There is a beautiful folk-saying in German referring to the mist that hangs over forests and trees in the early morning air being caused by *"Die Füchse kuchen Kaffee"* – "the foxes making coffee." Other variations of this saying include "the witches are making coffee", "the hares are making coffee", and *"Hexenküche"* the witch's kitchen (where all manner of magic may be cooking…). It seems that witches, hares and foxes are connected in both Germany and British folklore. The Danish also use similar inspiration, connecting brewing and morning mists: *"Mosekonen brygger"*, roughly translates to "the bog woman/the witch is brewing."

There is also a wonderful German children's book by Angela Sommer-Bodenburg from the early 1990s called *Wenn Die Füchse Kaffee Kochen*

(When the Foxes Make Coffee). I am sharing a short retelling of it here in English, and whilst I have changed elements to create my own version of the tale, it is very much inspired by Angela's beautiful book.

When The Foxes Make Coffee

A short adaptation of the story originally told by Angela Sommer-Bodenburg in her book Wenn Die Fusche Kaffee Kochen *(1992) and inspired by folklore.*

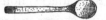

Evi loved visiting her aunt Ada in the country. Her little cottage sat within a large garden full of fruit trees and wildflowers that danced down into the valley that edged into the great trees of the Black Forest. Evi's mother had grown up in this cottage, and as they drove into the countryside, she told Evi that when they were younger she and Ada often searched for fairytale beings in the forest.

"And did you find them?" Evi asked excitedly.

Her mother winked and told her she would have to find out for herself as she dropped her off for a week's holiday at Aunt Ada's cottage.

On her first morning in the cottage, Evi rose early and looked out of her window. There she saw wisps of white sweeping from the end of the garden, through the valley and into the forest beyond. She'd never seen anything like this in the city! She ran down to her aunt to tell her of this strange sight. Ada laughed kindly. "That, my dear child, is the foxes. They are just making their morning coffee! They huddle around that pot of coffee at dawn, and we see the steam rising and winding its way through the trees and hanging in valley."

Well, Evi dearly wanted to see these fascinating foxes, so she decided that tomorrow she would go and meet them, and as is polite, she would take them a gift. So, she slipped into the pantry, took out a bag of coffee beans and put it in a little basket.

Evi tiptoed down the stairs very early the following day, grabbed the little basket, and slipped out the front door. She ran through the fruit trees, past crumbling stone walls and down into the valley and the forest's dense pine and birch trees. It was so early the moon still hung in the sky, and there was just a hint of the sun, which had not yet passed the horizon. There was no smoke to be seen anywhere; she wasn't sure where to start looking.

Evi began to feel her bravery and excitement ebb away a little…this was the Black Forest, after all, the place of witches, spirits, and hidden things, or so her book of fairy tales suggested. So, she sat on a tree stump, to think, and gather her courage.

All of a sudden, a little fox appeared between two silver birch trees. Evi leapt up and followed him quietly into a clearing in the trees. There in front of her, around a giant tree stump shaded by ancient trees was the little fox…as well as a middle-sized and a bigger fox, and betwixt them the giant tree stump was all set up for breakfast! A tablecloth of soft blue had been laid, and cups, saucers and plates were all neatly laid. They sensed her immediately, and all turned, six bright shining eyes upon her.

"Hello, my name is Evi," she stated clearly. "I wanted to meet you, so I brought you some coffee as a gift." She held out her basket to show the foxes.

Their foxy faces broke into wide smiles and they bid her to come closer!

Evi shuffled forwards, a little nervous. The foxes pulled out a chair, plumped pillows for her back and laid a blanket over her knees. They placed plates and cups before her.

"Please, join us! Friends are always welcome in the forest," the middle-sized fox said kindly.

The little fox ground the coffee beans and the bigger foxes swiftly brought wood and started a fire. Soon steam was rising from a kettle, hung over the fire from a branch. It rose high into the air in billowing white plumes. The white smoke!, Evi thought.

The boiling water was poured over the ground beans in the coffee pot, and the middle-sized fox took a deep sniff, and sighed happily. All the cups were filled with rich, dark coffee.

"What an aroma!" said the big fox.

"How delightful!" said the middle-sized fox.

"Cake time!" said the little fox. And the middle-sized fox brought out a large chocolate cake decorated with little sugar mice. A sumptuous breakfast indeed!

"How delicious!" said Evi, and indeed it was. She finished her slice then ate a second piece.

Feeling so warm and cosy and full of cake, Evi fell asleep under the trees. She awoke with a start, and tall shadow standing over her.

"I was worried about you," her aunt said seriously.

"But I came to meet the foxes!" Evi protested.

Ada laughed, surprised, "Dear girl, the story about the foxes is just a little tale!" said her aunt.

Evi looked around and saw that the tree stump was empty – cleared of cloth, cake and cups, even the little chairs had gone. Had she imagined everything?

But then the bag of coffee caught her eye. Nestled in foxgloves by a tree beside her, and it was empty... Ada picked up the empty bag and hugged Evi close, "Never mind, dear, you must have dropped the beans on the way."

Evi looked sadly down at the empty bag. But suddenly, a stream of white steam rising from the trees caught her eye. "Look!" she said, pointing over to the forest. "Do you see? The foxes are over there!"

"Oh, dear girl, that is just the fog that rises from the forest...though, I do recall when your mother and I were your age we imagined that there might be a witch cooking up magic in her steaming cauldron..." Ada said kindly and took Evi's hand.

But Evi knew better, "The foxes like my coffee so much they are having a second cup!"

Whisky

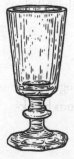

Wine, beer and cider all have their own folktales, and perhaps they have the closest likeness to the potion in the witch's cauldron: a bubbling liquid which with skill, knowledge and time transforms everyday ingredients into spirits capable of intoxication.

Whisky, *aqua vitae, uisge beatha* in Scottish Gaelic, "the water of life," is the potion I'll focus on here, as there's something so magical about it (as well as the fact that I adore a wee dram): the grain and the smoke, the wooden barrels, the alchemical process of distillation (and the resulting liquid gold…).

Witches and fairy folk run through many tales from the island of Islay, the southernmost of the Inner Hebrides islands, off the west coast of Scotland. Famous for its whisky distilleries: each distillery on Islay has its own amazing stories.

One of Scotland's greatest folklorists was born on this Island of Whisky in 1822: John Francis Campbell of Islay, known as the "lamplighter and storyteller." He was heir to the Isle of Islay, but he never came into this inheritance as the estate was sold. His passion lay in collecting Western Highlands' folklore, drawn from oral accounts. He travelled extensively, recording tales, ballads, songs, charms and anecdotes which were published in four volumes of *Popular Tales of the West Highlands* in the mid-1800s.

The stories in this section have been gathered over the years, thanks to the wonderful distillery reps at whisky tasting events and distillery tours, books of whisky legends, wise barmen, and trips to the Highlands. "The Fairy Queen" and "Angel of Islay" are drawn from stories found in *Whisky Legends of Islay* by Robin Laing and *The Inner Hebrides and their Legends* by Otta F. Swire, with some extra embellishments from myself, other storytellers and whisky fans along the way! Just weeks before submitting the final draft of this book, I settled down to read Dr. Sharon Blackie's *If Women Rose Rooted* and nearly dropped it when on the first page was another version of the Fairy Queen story, this one featuring the queen of the *Aos Sí*.[*] So, I am now aware of versions of the story from both Irish and Scottish folklore of fairy queens, feasts and of women being the ones who truly understood the 'Otherworld' and wisdom from it. I imagine there are many similar stories surrounding the fairy hills of all the Celtic lands, but perhaps the golden flagons of whisky are a unique feature of Scottish fairy lore.

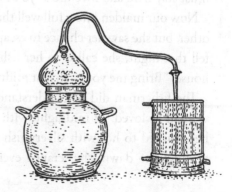

[*]   The mythical Irish fairy race.

The Angel from Islay

A rich whisky merchant owned a distillery on Islay. His house was fine, with a large garden that grew flowers and looked over the fishing town and harbour. He dreamed of starting a family to pass down the distillery to his heirs one day, so he went about finding a wife.

All about the island he travelled, seeking a fair and beautiful woman. He had been around the island twice but had found no woman right for him. He had almost given up hope as he returned to his house overlooking the harbour. There he came across a poor fisherman and his beautiful fiancée. The woman had golden amber hair like a glass of whisky held up to the sun and deep dark brown eyes like charred oak barrels. The merchant was smitten. Being a businessman, our whisky merchant was ruthless and single-minded, and with no thought to the couple's previous engagement, he promptly offered the young woman's parents such a fine dowry for her hand that a new match was made. The whisky merchant married his young bride. Her heart broke for her lost love with the fisherman and she was filled with anger that these choices had been made for her.

Time passed and she spoke not one word to the merchant, or to anyone. She sat at the window of her large house and watched her fisherman toil at his work at the harbour. She watched the light of his boat as he sailed out each night as the moon rose. She would weep and whisper his name.

The merchant grew frustrated. Had he not offered his bride untold riches? Why did she not love him? So he, being a man of the world, made a deal with her: "If you can steal my soul by morning, I shall be turned to stone by the Devil himself, and you will be free. But should you fail, you must stay here and love me as you love your fisher fellow."

Now our maiden knew full well that no one could be forced to love another, but she saw her chance to escape and took it regardless. As darkness fell that night, she called to her fisherman from the gardens of her fine house, "Bring me your catch at midnight, my love, and I will set us free."

The fisherman did not understand, but he did as he was told for the woman he loved. At midnight, with the full moon high in the night sky, he returned to her with silvery fish that shone in the moonlight. From midnight to dawn, she scraped every scale from every fish into a bowl and, with such labour that only love can provoke, sewed thousands upon thousands of shining scales into a gown and a pair of great gossamer wings. As dawn broke the next morning, the merchant walked out of his front door and was met by the sight of her, so shining she was, the dawn light lit her aglow, he thought her an angel. He fell to his knees and offered up his soul to the angel.

Our angel bride lowered her wings, and the merchant saw the morning light upon her face, and he smiled sadly. He had made his promise. She leaned down and placed a gentle kiss upon his forehead and whispered, "Thank you," as he turned to stone, still kneeling on the ground.

She ran to her fisherman love, and they lived happily ever after, filling the house of the merchant with laughter and children. They kept a keen eye over the distillery with their happy family. When, after many years, her life came to a peaceful end, her sons took ownership of the distillery, and she became the great angel who looks down over all the distilleries of Islay, sampling the whisky that rises through the barrels, the angel's share of the whisky. She does her part to make sure that every single angel gets their share of whisky, and of love!

The Angel's Share, and the Devil's Cut

The angel's share is a feature of whisky maturation. Scotch whisky must be matured in oak barrels for at least three years. But oak barrels are porous, and they absorb liquid over time, so some of the spirit that goes into a cask will be absorbed into the wood. And a smaller proportion will travel right through the wood grain and out into the atmosphere – up to the angels in what is called "the angel's share." A cask that is very old could be half empty by the time it is bottled, which is one reason why older whisky tends to be more expensive. The whisky left absorbed in the wood, on the other hand, is called the Devil's cut; I like to imagine the Devil cracking open each barrel and sucking from the staves like barbeque ribs. Some distilleries have worked out how to extract this Devil's cut to put into special edition bottles…but it would take a braver soul than I to deprive the Devil of his cut of whisky!

Under the fairy hill at Ardbeg, lives the Fairy Queen. Knowing that life could be difficult for the women of the Scottish islands, she sent out some very special invitations to the land of humans. She sent messages by sea, carried by seals and otters; by land, with the sure-footed deer and brown hare; carried on the winds in the beaks of oystercatchers, puffins, corncrake and curlew; and clutched in little furry claws of the ptarmigans. This invitation was for all the women to join her at a sumptuous feast under the fairy hill, so that she may share some of her fairy wisdom with them. For, like Kerridwen and her cauldron, in the world of fairies, it is women who hold the cup from which wisdom is dispensed. On receiving their invitations some women were intrigued, others wary, but many arrived on a bright and breezy day to Islay, and the harbour was filled with boats with sails of every colour. And streams of women hiked from every corner of Islay's shores.

As these women approached the hill, a great door opened and they were warmly welcomed inside. The Fairy Queen's hall was resplendent with tapestries of finest weaving, exquisite colours extracted from plants: purple of every shade, darkest hues of blackberries, reds, oranges from rowan and rich reds from raspberries. But the most beautiful shades were those of green – the brightest, lightest greens drawn from the youngest shoots of spring to the deepest darkest hues of winter holly. There were lights aplenty: candles burned on the tables and jars held merrily dancing fireflies. Crystal chandeliers and glowing lamps lit the hall from above, prisms caught beams of sunlight from skylights and cast rainbow colours upon the floor.

A fabulous banquet was laid out on platters of carved slate. There were goblets of turned wood, bowls of mother of pearl shell and delicate glasses shaped like the cairns built on the highest mountain peaks to honour Scottish warriors.

The Fairy Queen made a grand entrance. Some say the fairies were once goddesses, and the Queen looked like a regal earth goddess in her gown of every shade of the island – greens, browns, stony greys and ocean blues. She bade the party to sit, and the fairies served them a sumptuous feast. They chatted merrily together as they ate and drank.

After a delicious, sweet course of honeyed oatcakes and blueberries, the Fairy Queen rose and clapped her hands for silence. She told the women her reason for inviting them here was that they may leave with more answers than questions. She wanted them to pass on the knowledge of the fairy folk to their daughters and granddaughters as well as those too afraid to visit the hill that day.

She lifted a golden flagon from the table, telling them all that this vessel held the precious golden liquid that was the distilled knowledge of the world: a wisdom gathered in the elemental journey of the liquid made of earth, air, fire, and water. It had been acquired over countless generations of fairy women and was guarded by the Fairy Queen herself. The flagon was large, and when passed around, each woman filled their delicate glasses with the golden liquid. There was plenty to go round.

The Queen raised her glass and made a toast in her fairy tongue, and all the women raised their glasses and drank. The liquid had a fiery touch and a warmth that trickled through their hearts and bellies. They felt a warm glow radiate through them, a calm and a confidence that permeated their bodies, heart and minds. Silence fell. There were no more questions, for all questions had been answered: the water of life had told them all the secrets of being and knowledge of the fairies.

After warm farewells and thanks to the hostess, the women prepared to leave this beautiful feast and return home. When they came out into the sunshine, they were illuminated with light from within and above. They sought to spread the gift of wisdom from the golden whisky flagon of the Fairy Queen.

Whisky, Women and Royal Witches

Throughout Europe in the 1500s cities banned domestic *aqua vitae* production, (which was the blanket term for these nascent distilled alcoholic beverages – so included early and rustic versions of whisky and vodka). This ban stopped many women from making spirits and also from much healing work. Just as alewives had been condemned as witches, some accusers claimed *aqua vitae* turned people into demons, and those who used it were witches. If *aqua vitae* was found in someone's dwellings and it was not prescribed by a doctor, this was enough evidence to accuse them of practising witchcraft.

In 1418 Joan of Navarre, Queen of England and second wife of Henry IV of England, was imprisoned and accused of witchcraft and sorcery. Apparently, the evidence against her included possession of *aqua vitae*.[12] While she was accused, she was never tried, and she was eventually set free from a rather luxurious imprisonment to live a quiet, comfortable life. Later, in 1441, Eleanor Cobham, Duchess of Gloucester, confessed to practising alchemical magic after she was found in possession of a vial of *aqua vitae*. She had most likely obtained this from the wise woman she employed named Margery Jourdemayne – known as "the Witch of Eye," renowned as a skilled maker of potions, folk medicines and charms. Both were accused of plotting to kill Henry VI by magical means. The Duchess denied most of the charges but admitted to procuring potions from Margery, in an effort to help her conceive. Margery was burned at the stake as a heretic, and Eleanor was forced to renounce her heresies and witchcraft and was imprisoned for life. So royal life too had its fair share of witchcraft accusations (and alcohol).

It is possible that angry neighbours may have accused female whisky distillers of being witches, however most *aqua vitae*-related witch convictions came from women brewing folk medicine remedies. In 1623 in Scotland a woman called Janet Ross was executed for (among other things) prescribing a patient with a fever an egg with a little *aqua vitae* and pepper.

Widely used in American folk medicine, whiskey also plays a role in contemporary American folk magic. A piece of agar (a type of seaweed) is put into a jar of whiskey and allowed to soak. This is done to attract "good spirits."[13]

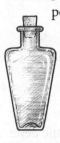

During America's Prohibition in the 1920s, whisky could be legally imported because it was considered a medicine. A prescription from your doctor for medical whisky was one of the only ways to get your hands on a drink in that era. Even today it is still connected to healing. In moderation, whisky can dilate blood vessels, and like all alcohol, has a mild anaesthetic and antiseptic effect, which might explain why Hot Toddies are still such a popular home remedy for cold and flu symptoms. However, too much alcohol or an addiction to it, can kill you: the paradox of many herbs and medicines than can be beneficial but in the wrong doses, deadly.

So just a dram, to your good health. The word "dram" or drachm is a term originally used for an apothecary's weight, which now we use almost exclusively for whisky. Another nod to its connection with medicine.

The Whisky Named After a Boat, Named After a Witch, Named After a Nightie...

This is the story of Tam O'Shanter, an old Scottish legend that was later turned into a poem by Robert Burns. I know it's a bit of a curveball, but hey, witches and whisky are involved in this little tale (and tail) of the Cutty Sark, which is a boat, and a whisky...and they are both named for a witch's night time attire!

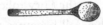

We meet our protagonist Tam after an enjoyable evening drinking at a pub. He's been boozing on strong ale and making merry. Tam starts his journey home on his faithful horse, Meg. But on his way, what should he see but a coven of witches dancing around a bonfire in a churchyard. He is quite bewitched by the sight of Nannie Dee, a beautiful witch wearing nought but a small nightdress – a 'cutty sark,' which is an old Scottish name for a short nightdress. Our enamoured Tam calls out to Nanny, "Weel done, Cutty-sark!" in his approval of her tiny attire. But Nanny and the witches are not happy, and Nanny gives chase to this drunkard cat-caller and his horse.

Tam heads for the river because, according to some folklore, witches cannot cross running water. They make it just in time, but as they are crossing, Nannie reaches out and grabs Meg's tail, which comes away in her hand.

One day, many years later, a Scottish boat designer suggested that they name a brand-new tea clipper after the Cutty Sark of the story, perhaps a challenge to the legend that witches cannot cross running water. The Cutty Sark clipper became well-known as one of the fastest ships of its day. And Nannie Dee has pride of place as the boat's figurehead, with Meg's tail still grasped in her hand. You can still see the Cutty Sark, which is in permanent dock in Greenwich, London. And as for the whisky, it was named after the boat, not the witch, as far as I can tell...

What Whisky Can't Cure... Irish Whiskey Lore

An rud nach leigheasann im ná uisce beatha níl an leigheas air.

"What butter or whiskey doesn't cure, cannot be cured."

Irish proverb

I'm not going to delve too deeply into the debate of who distilled it first, the Scots or the Irish, but by 1405, whisky/*aqua vitae*/*uisge beatha* was appearing in written records. Some stories involve monks sharing secrets of distillation from the East, traders bringing grains from Africa and Asia.

In some Irish folklore, they say the fairy folk, the Tuatha Dé Danann, are fallen angels, and the place they fall becomes their domain, creating fairies of forest, mountain, ocean and land. So perhaps the *clurichaun* fell into a whiskey* barrel...

The *clurichaun* is a mischievous soul known for his love of drinking whiskey and his tendency to haunt pubs, wine cellars, breweries and distilleries. Such is his fondness for alcohol, he is very rarely seen without a dram or beer in his hand. Cousin of the better-known leprechaun, the *clurichaun* is more likely to be at the end of the rainbow not with a pot of gold but a tankard of beer or perhaps a golden dram.

Clurichauns can pass through keyholes to invade homes and wine cellars. Being loyal creatures, they endeavour to protect their property and the lives of those within it. They tend to attach themselves to noble families (as they are the ones with the best wine cellars), but such is their appetite for boozing that they can bring speedy ruin to the homeowner. *Clurichauns* are said to fly through the air on rushes similar to witches. And also, like witches, disgruntled *clurichauns* are often blamed for your milk turning sour, family and livestock illness, and eggs made rotten, as well, of course, as booze cupboards cleared out, so offerings of food and drink should be laid out to appease them.

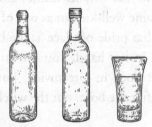

---

* In Scotland it is spelt whisky, in Ireland, whiskey.

SECTION TWO SUMMARY

To truly understand a group of people, you need to look at the culture of everyone, not just a select few. Jokes, sayings, legends, superstitions – they're all part of a folklore that we are continually creating into the present day. The images, archetypes and themes we find in folk and fairy tales resonate with a universal consciousness or collective unconscious that ensures the continued popularity of these age-old stories, their characters, structures and meanings. One of these themes is, of course, as one of our most universal physical needs – food.

Our shared cultural creations of food and folklore show us what we have found meaningful over the centuries, perhaps because it makes us laugh, offers us hope, or outlines hard lessons. Stories of the witch, the Devil and fairy folk play a large part in the rich folklore of food. Connected to some of its vital magical and medicinal properties, as well as salves, tinctures, and remedies which are passed down, and the stories continued.

In each culture, we find stories within stories, echoes of other tales, hands held over countries and county lines, smiles of recognition over oceans – a collective memory that the princesses with long shining hair would be kind, that talking animals should be listened to carefully (as useful guides or tricksters), and that you should always take care when walking into the woods and eating the supper of others without permission, as well as always being generous and mindful with food.

As the world turns, much will be forgotten in time, but stories, folklore, magic are things we can pass on and share. Language itself is deep and ancient magic: we can use poetry to cast spells, offer story as a magical art, and use it as a vehicle of myth. Folk and fairy tales can be a way of discussing worlds we have come out of, and perhaps, the worlds we want to live in.

Words woven into story can create surprise, wonder, meaning that stays with us. The symbols, imagery, and associations we find in stories may enable us to understand ourselves, each other, and our communities better, and perhaps to see a little more magic and wonder in the world.

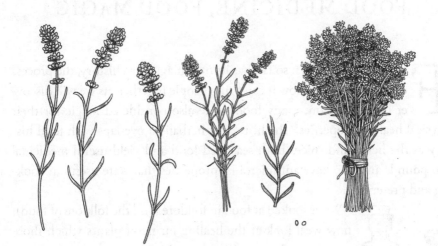

SECTION THREE

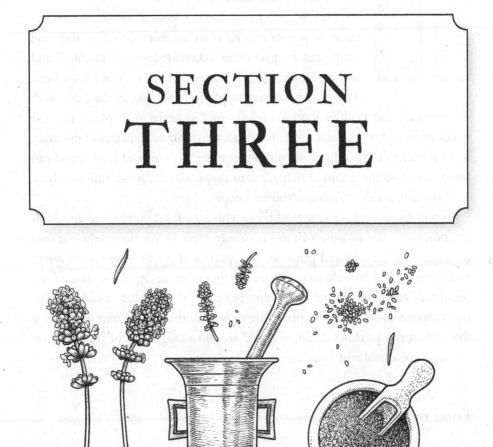

FOOD MEDICINE, FOOD MAGIC

F ood, as we have seen so far, has its own magic – its history, the process of creating it, and how it can bring people together. As we will discover in this section, many foods were also considered magic for their physical healing properties. The history of herbalism overlaps with food history as the herbs and spices both seasoned food and yield useful medicinal compounds and also have antimicrobial properties that were useful in cooking and preserving.

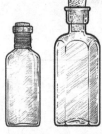

We've looked at food in folklore (and the folklore of food), now we'll look at the healing magic of plants which those stories and superstitions may hint at.

Power is present in food, whether we choose to acknowledge it or not. Kitchen witchery, cooking, and food magic can be part of an acknowledgement of this. Food and magic work in all manner of ways. As we'll see here, there is the capacity to promote healing in the body with whole foods and healthy foods, carefully picked herbs and spices. But the magic of food does not end there. Food can transport us to places of memory, to joyful celebrations, times of coming together to cook and feast. Food can bring out excitement and anticipation to revisit our favourite dining tables, our favourite meals with our favourite people.

We will discover many stories of those who used food for magical and healing purposes. The folklore of food is closely woven with the medicinal uses of plants. The healing and poisonous properties of plants were secrets learnt and often shared by informal means. Many ended up in the realms of superstition, relics of charms and prescriptions of the witches, and countless superstitions connected with plants are to be found at the present day. I hope that the stories in this section will help to move magic out of the cauldron and into the world and your day.

Food for Thought

Whether you talk to a witch, a Buddhist, a neuroscientist, a doctor, a Christian or a casual meditation fan, the power of thought – whether that is intention, spell work, manifestation, visualisation or prayer is both possible and very real.* We know that thoughts have the ability to create change, which for many is the essence of magic and witchcraft. But while most people are aware and believe in the influence of the mind, they perhaps don't care to dwell on it too much. You may think of food magic as intentions and mindfulness creating changes in yourself and those around you, or herbs and food having a physical effect on your physiology, or in any way that inspires you.

Part of food magic is about connecting to the lore of food and the energies that are contained in the food. Every time you prepare a meal you have the opportunity to create small positive changes: for love, health, happiness, and protection. In cooking, you begin with basic ingredients, which are then turned into something nourishing and beneficial in some way. I'm not going to say every meal has to be prepared with intentions and each ingredient selected for its symbolism or magical properties. Few of us have the energy to do that all the time. But, each meal, snack, drink has the *potential* to be an act of magic, maybe not a full ritual or act of witchcraft – but a tiny spark of gratitude, a celebration that magically changes the food you prepare. You can choose to make an offering to the Earth Mother by crumbling a corner of your sandwich on the ground for a pigeon, or by offering a splash of wine for our "noble spirit," as the ancient Greeks did. This is not so much seeking out magic from dark corners and esoteric texts, as seeing the magic in the light of the everyday.

Some of us may never have the ability to see the future in apple pips (although many would say it is an innate skill that can be nurtured), but all of us can create a meal in our kitchens or over a fire, no matter how simple. We get to embody the Kitchen Witch here and now. We can all grind peppercorns and break star anise, slice ginger and stir honey into tea...these small reminders that we are all capable of magic and that everyday actions can be magical.

---

* Thoughts have power: from the placebo effect to the rather ominous sounding voodoo death phenomenon (coined around 1942 where, based on field studies, sometimes connected to a curse you believe to be upon you, it is possible to die purely from the belief that you will).

The Magic of Food – Alexis Prior, nutritionist

For me, the magic of food is that, simply put, everything we eat is what we become. Our entire being, including bones, skin, muscle, immune system, hormones, heart, brain, are all created from our food and drink. Even our moods and feelings are influenced by our diet.

When we eat healthful food, we give ourselves the basics for abundant physical and mental health. When we eat poor quality, processed foods in large amounts, we can't build a healthy body or mind.

Of course, we can go further. Everything we consume or are exposed to also affects our health, including what's in our environment that we breathe and absorb through our skin, and what we consume mentally via relationships, media, or our internal thoughts. But food is the one thing that gives us the actual raw materials to build a wonderful healthy body.

But not all food can do this.

The magic comes from whole, unadulterated food. Food that doesn't come in a box with a list of chemicals. Whole, natural food contains a myriad of wonderful nutrients. It's not just a case of carbohydrate, protein or fat. It's not just vitamins and minerals. Plants contain hundreds if not thousands of complex phytochemicals that support our immune system, protect our beautiful, beneficial bacteria and enhance our physical and mental being. It's not each individual component of food but all of these factors together, working in harmony, in a complex web of relationships that make the difference. The whole is greater than the sum of the parts. If we isolate ingredients, we can lose the magic.

I love the concept that food is information. This goes beyond the nutrients in the food and considers the effect of the contents of the food on our bodies. For example, foods such as sugar, refined carbohydrates and poor quality fats put our body on high alert and in an inflammatory state which can lead to poor health. Whereas whole colourful plant foods, certain spices and omega-3 fatty acids have an anti-inflammatory effect in our bodies and promote good health.

Let's go even further, though. How we eat our food can also create magic. Compare an egg sandwich from a garage, eaten in your car whilst driving up the motorway, with a lovingly prepared poached egg on toast, eaten with friends for a leisurely brunch on a Sunday morning. Same ingredients, but a totally different experience. One is mindlessly shovelling fuel. The other is love, care, appreciation and connection.

So yes, food can be magic: simple, unadulterated natural food eaten in a mindful, appreciative way. Ideally, with loved ones!

CUNNING FOLK

Once, in every rural (and many an urban) home without access to a doctor (which was many), women were responsible for the healing, as well as nourishment, and care of both their family and animals. Women who would have held no official titles, women who faced incredible challenges of raising children, feeding, cooking, preserving, weaving the best they could with the knowledge passed down to them, and for which they received little or no recognition. Grandmothers might divine fortunes, treat ailments, and create charms for healing. Midwives helped both bring new life into the world and lay out the dead. They held respected positions in an age when women otherwise had little status.

In medieval times, living conditions were poor and could be cut short by minor injuries, such as infections. Doctors were scarce and expensive, and early medicinal practices such as bloodletting and amputations could actually make things worse. For members of Europe's lower classes, local healers were often the only option. They were highly respected, sought out and consulted for healing and for answers. In the British Isles, we knew these people as "cunning folk" – professional practitioners (both male and female) of folk magic from the medieval period onward who charged for their skills and services. They might also, depending on who you spoke to, be called, either by themselves or others – witches, pellars,* wise women, healers and magicians.

The history of folk medicine is entwined with myths, folk tales, fairy tales, and the homespun magic of these cunning folk. The cunning one was someone who would listen and offer magical practices and wise words to deal with

* A Cornish term for witch.

all manner of everyday troubles, drawing from many practices and modalities. Each had their own areas of expertise, and they may well have used a mix of practices including spells, incantations, rituals, and skills in empathy and intuition. They were sought out to cure illness, find lost objects, and remove curses or malevolent forces imposed by witches or other supposed evildoers.

WYRTCUNNING

In Old English "wyrtcunning" means plant knowledge. In Saxon times, someone skilled in wyrtcunning would be called on, just a doctor is today.

Wyrt or *wort,* meaning a plant and its bounty, is still found in the common, country or folk names of many herbs and hedgerow plants: St. John's wort, mugwort, bishop's wort, dragonwort, liverwort, lungwort and bladderwort. These last three got their names from the shape of their leaves, rather than their curative properties…whereas birthwort, motherwort, feverwort and bruisewort got their names from their medicinal uses. Interestingly, wort is also the name for the sweet liquid extracted from the mash (ground malt and grain) process during the brewing of beer or whisky. Both uses of the word date back to before the twelfth century. *Cunning* meant a skill or knowledge, and you could liken it to modern day areas of study: herbology or herbalism. This was very much everyday magic and healing. At this time, it wasn't a case of whether people 'believed' in it, it was simply what was there, a trust in the land and nature.

Cunning Folk, Witches and Fairies

Witches, fairies, and cunning folk are woven together in many historical accounts. The following are just some from the south of England.

In 1566 John Walsh, a cunning man from Dorsetshire, said fairies helped his healing work. He was accused, but found not guilty, of witchcraft. Ann Jeffries, in Cornwall around 1640, reported that she was visited by fairies who gave her the ability to cure the sick and gifted her with clairvoyance. She was never formally tried for witchcraft but was still held in Bodmin Jail, records say, without food or water for three months. She survived, apparently, because the fairies bought her food in the cold damp prison, so she lived on honey, dew drops and fairy pasties. Certainly, some forces allowed her to survive so long in terrible conditions. In 1619 cunning woman Joan Willimot from Goadsby* also said fairies helped her detect and cure victims of harmful magic; she also had various familiar spirits.

It would have been very common to see cunning folk in villages in England in the 1500s and 1600s. But, as the fear of magic grew slowly over the centuries, working with magic, especially openly in this way, became dangerous. At the peak of the witch hunts in the British Isles, it was dancing that fine line between who was thought to be using magic for 'good' and who was not, and these cunning folk could be identified as witches themselves. Some witches were cunning folk, and some cunning folk cast spells and charms against witches, and some cunning folk were accused of being witches by disgruntled clients. It's a muddle when so many folk medicine traditions all get bundled together! So, whilst many were well-respected, the profession was not without its dangers (maybe more so, for the more unscrupulous practitioners).

Cunning folk and witches alike used everyday objects – stones, feathers, sticks, bones, wax, bottles and anything that came readily to hand in the kitchen or farmstead. This is the ancient wisdom of our ancestors, once passed down and then developed by a lifetime of study by those seeking to learn the arts of cunning craft and witchery. And though few women were accorded adequate status for their work, this expertise formed a pattern for women's lives for thousands of years.

But power shifts began, as knowledge became something considered 'owned' by male experts and could only be passed on through academic institutions. Those seeking to follow traditional or alternative paths were dismissed as uneducated, naive or even dangerous. Women's knowledge became mocked as old wives tales, notions, intuitions, fancies – as it still is today.

---

* Joan Willimot also had the dubious honour of appearing on the cover of a witch trial pamphlet, *The Wonderful Discoverie of the Witchcrafts of Margaret and Philip Flower*, 1619 in a woodcut print, alongside Anne Baker and Ellen Greene, with a variety of familiars. All the women are elderly, blind and/or walk with the aid of sticks, which tells you a lot about the kind of women accused and the stereotypes held about anyone who was considered 'different'. These pamphlets of the witch trials were sold cheaply and no doubt many people enjoy the scandal and fantastical stories of evil deeds and devilish mischief. But this also caused a perpetuation of these images of what a witch looked like and fed suspicion.

CANTRIPS AND CHARMS

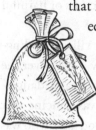

Many of the practices of witchcraft connect so closely to healing because that is exactly what it was for, as early medicine. Lack of knowledge of the human body and its functions brought an element of mystery and magic which surrounded the subject of medicine, and someone who could successfully treat disease was regarded by many as possessing of otherworldly powers, which could be painted as a good or a bad thing depending on someone's biases. Until the practice of medicine came to be established upon scientific principles, the care of the sick largely fell upon women, who became both nurse and physician. Something they would later be condemned for.

The witch-hunting book *Malleus Maleficarum*[*] focused on women healers. According to the book, the women most likely to be witches were midwives (along with adulteresses and fornicators.) As far as the author of the book was concerned, if a woman dared to cure without having studied, then she was definitely a witch. Of course, this refers to studying at medical schools that forbid women, so this was a 'no-win' situation. The cunning woman or midwife would have studied in the kitchen of her foremothers and in the hedges and woodland floor. But obviously, this was lost on the witchfinders. Women's knowledge was derided, ignored, not just her skill with herbs and tinctures, but curative methods of healing touch, connection and intuition, the very earliest form of talking therapy and counselling. It was the empathy, caring, and healing skills of women that ultimately worked against them. Benevolent, compassionate skills and arts were misunderstood by the patriarchy and became twisted by fear. They still are.

So, whilst some of the European witches were explicitly described as healers or midwives, most historians and scribes of the early modern period largely ignored the role of women in the providing of medical services or dismissed them with belittling terms, their value reduced and dismissed. It was incredible that men could both deride the skills of witches and healing women and yet use similar methods themselves. You can see it in the *Malleus Maleficar-*

---

[*] Although at the time, some people (quite rightly) thought the author Heinrich Kramer was a bit of a crank and condemned his extreme practices, the *Malleus* remains one of the most well-known witch hunting texts, and it illustrates the extreme biases held by witch hunters.

um, where it seems that it's not the *method* but the *sex* of the one administering it that separates superstition from science. Of male doctors it is clear that, "although some of their remedies seem to be vain and superstitious cantrips and charms...everyone must be trusted in his profession."

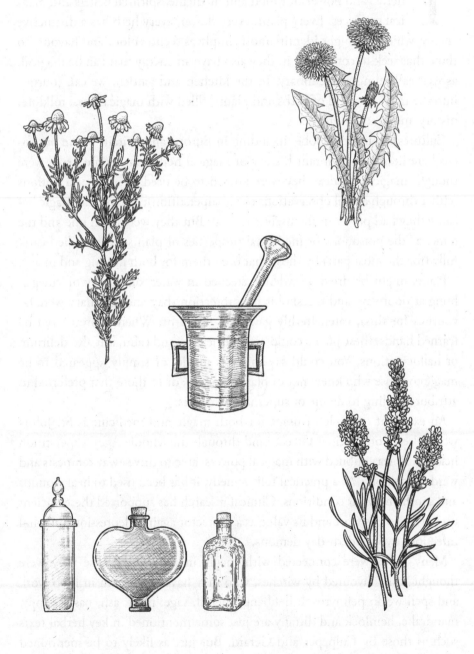

MAGICAL HERBALISM

Through the development of civilisations, we've relied on plants, herbs, and flowers for food and medicine, spiritual beliefs and magical practices. Every plant, every flower, every herb has a distinctive energy, which we might identify most simply as scent, colour and flavour. To those that seek to connect to it, they also have an energy that can be magical, as well as healing and culinary. In the kitchen and garden, we can journey into the magical world of herbs and plants, filled with magical uses, folklore, history and practical magic.

Cultures around the globe, including in Europe and Britain where our focus here lies, have a vibrant history of magical herbalism. Some herbs were thought magical because they were known to be used in spells and potions (either through actual observations or via superstition); others held magic because they had power in themselves to heal. But they were often one and the same, as the poisonous or medicinal properties of plants were studied carefully (for the most part) by those that used them for both healing and magic.

Plants might be dried, powdered, steeped in water, oil, honey or vinegar, hung at doorways and thresholds for protection (bay and rosemary were favourites for this), eaten freshly gathered, or burnt. When administered by learned hands, these plants could conjure healing and calm, but also delirium or hallucinations. You could say this was magic, or simply appeared to be magic to those who knew not of plants' powers, or to those that preferred to attribute healing to divine or supernatural causes.

An excellent example of usage for both magic and medicine is St. John's wort. Used from ancient Greece, and through the Middle Ages, superstition held that it was imbued with magical powers: able to drive away tempests and ward off demons. As a practical folk-remedy, it has been used to heal wounds and soothe nervous conditions. Clinical research has supported these ancient uses of St. John's wort and its value as a protector against depression and viral infection, two modern-day demons.

Many herbs were connected with magic in folklore because they were thought to be favoured by witches, who may have used them in herb work and spell work: pennyroyal, henbane, chervil, sage, mint, ash, basil, poppy, mandrake, hemlock and dittany are just some mentioned in key herbal texts such as those by Culpeper and Gerard. But just as likely to be mentioned were herbs thought to repel witches: valerian, elder, angelica, and all yellow flowers, as they were thought to be connected to the sun (based on the assumption that light repels witches, who preferred the dark night apparently). This possibly may be as they were less likely to use those plants in healing. Many plants ended up with superstitions attached as both friend and foe of the witch, depending on areas and local lore. The only true curators perhaps, of the most favoured magical herbs were the witches themselves, and perhaps they would have known better than to announce them publicly.

It is a wonderful image to think of all witches working in their beautiful cottage gardens and gathering herbs and berries from hedgerows – but many a witch worked in the grit and gravel of overcrowded cities and towns, perhaps barely working with herbs at all. Luckily today wherever we live we are more able to access nature and bring it into our homes with even just a simple houseplant or windowsill herb garden.

Cunning Belladonna

Not all connections between plants and magic were positive. Some of the earliest imagery of witchcraft connected witches with herbs like *Atropa belladonna,* commonly known as belladonna or deadly nightshade. Used by cunning women as a muscle relaxant and pain reliever, alkaloids from belladonna are still be found in some medicines; but it is also very toxic. It was favoured by witches of myth like Medea and, more recently, the Owens sisters of *Practical Magic.*

Belladonna's use by healers is one connection to the witch, but also the dual nature of the plant itself is perhaps another: to some she is *bella donna,* from the Latin/Italian for "beautiful lady," to others she is deadly, viewed with suspicion. Whichever your view, it's certainly wise to treat her with respect. The name belladonna originally came from ancient Rome when women used to apply the juice of the berries to their eyes in order to cause their pupils to dilate (a glamour potion many died for). And the full name of *Atropa belladonna* is in reference to Atropos, one of the Three Fates in Greek mythology who snipped the thread of life. Powerful imagery for a powerful plant!

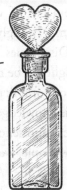

Magic – High and Low

Women who worked as healers had a tradition of excellent knowledge of plants for fertility and healing, intoxication and magic. They were the primary caretakers of knowledge of natural and home remedies. "Home remedies" is another term that has come to mean 'lesser' – primal, or rudimentary today. But this was once, simply, the way of daily life. It was what saved lives and maintained health for the majority of humanity. Those who practiced ceremonial and ritual magic, especially the more academic classes, often called their own path "high magic" and referred to this magic of the home as "low magic." But as Patricia Talesco reminds us in her book, *The Kitchen Witch's Cookbook* (1994), "Simplicity does not imply weakness, nor do fancy rituals ensure dynamic magical results. Neither approach is better or more powerful, they are simply different means for different individuals or circumstances."

We can still find remnants of ancient healing work. Archaeological digs can uncover possible clues as to how a culture used herbs, in what is known as archaeobotany – archaeology that specifically studies plant remains to explore how people used plants in the past. We know that herbs were used in rituals of brewing, healing, birth, magic and death in our history. Archaeological discoveries can show us a more personal story, such as remnants of plants buried with the dead. Traces of meadowsweet have been found in Neolithic burial sites in areas of Wales and Scotland. This herb has long been used to both sweeten mead, soothe pain and induce deep sleep, perhaps in burial it was a floral invitation to 'rest in peace.'

Excavations in Sweden offer us precious clues as to the use of plants and herbs in Viking age Scandinavia. The herb motherwort was found in the stomachs of women buried with infants, which, along with its common name, strongly suggests it was used by midwives and in the birthing process.

Discoveries such as this are so important because many common herbs might not be mentioned in any written sources. This is very much a consideration for folk practices and especially the practices of women and midwives – this knowledge didn't always make the written sources of higher-class doctors, men, and scholars. It is only amongst the remains of the settlements, around the people, we find suggestions of the magic of herbs used to heal and soothe in daily life. And as, over time, beliefs about plants turned from everyday magic and a lived reality into the realm of folklore and superstitions, our cultural knowledge may have diminished.

But embers of this knowledge still exist, glowing in the hearths, passed down through generations. And in modern movements such as our guide on this journey, the Kitchen Witch, we may start seeing a re-emergence and a reclaiming of magical ritual and higher connection with plants. From the simplest acts of infusing herbs in water or using them in cooking, you are altering the state of both, creating something entirely new, charged with energy from both herb and healer in a potent magical herbalism all of your own.

HERBWIVES

In modern-day witchery, you might call yourself a Kitchen Witch or Green Witch to identify your areas of passion or expertise. From the Middle Ages and well into modern times in England, the commodity women created and sold could be part of her identity and name, and you may meet them regularly at market: applewives, fishwives, oysterwives and herbwives. There was seemingly no end to variations, in a poem by Keats called "Over the Hill, Over the the Dale" we meet "ginger-bread wives," and in an essay, Francis Bacon spoke of "Strawberrie wives, that laid two or three great strawberries at the mouth of their pot, and all the rest were little ones," (a sales technique still in use today!). These 'wives' were often denounced as "unruly," frequently painted as swindlers: loud-mouthed and untrustworthy (an insult we still use today in English, calling a woman a fishwife if they are loud and coarse).

Herbwives would use a variety of plants from their own gardens and wild places, the hedges and verges of country lanes to make their living selling bundles of fresh herbs and often preparations of infusions, healing salves and folk medicines. Traditional herbal remedies were created for domestic use, culinary and medicinal purposes, such as for cleaning surfaces, flavouring stock, food preservation or as a soothing balm for burns or sores. Bundles of herbs were often used not just for cooking, but for decoration and good luck.

Buy Rue! Buy Sage! Buy Mint!
   Buy Rue, Sage and Mint, a farthing a bunch!

As thro' the fields she bends her way,
Pure nature's work discerning;
So you should practice every day,
To trace the fields of learning.

Charles Hindley, *A History of the Cries of London Ancient and Modern* (1876)

In larger cities, the medical hierarchy would have seen male physicians trained at colleges in the top tier of respectability, then barbers performing minor surgeries like dental work, and apothecaries in the middle, and these 'unruly' women may be found at the bottom, including midwives and herbwives.

Sometimes one and the same, herbwives could also be midwives or help in childbirth. Some herbs are known to ease labour, and common issues like infection might be treated with plants like garlic and yarrow, whilst cuts and scrapes would be cleaned and perhaps wrapped in burdock leaves to promote healing.

The herbwife was generally well respected in rural communities, but in both city and country the herbwife walked that fine line between being seen as a healer or a witch, especially in areas high in witch accusations, like Scotland and Germany. If she employed charms, lost too many patients, or had a brash manner (to name a few of many risky behaviours) she could be accused as a witch, lose her profession and very possibly her life.

HEALING WORDS

Stories are essential to the healing practices of many (if not all) native cultures. The words and the telling can be healing as well as the knowledge they contain. A legacy of herbal remedies handed down would have been part of the informal education of the household. The type of herb one would use would depend on what your medicine was for: to reduce inflammation, boost the immune system, calm the nerves, or support digestion. And there would be known recipes for each of these remedies that also included prayers or charms as part of the process.

Anyone who saw the bounty available in the land may well have used stories not only to preserve and pass on information about the medicinal properties of plants but also as a medium of communicating with the spirits of the plants themselves. Many similar practices can be seen the world over with shamans, witch doctors and medicine men and women who form a personal relationship with the plants they heal with. We are back at that idea of magic being about participating and connecting. Some people sing and talk to their plants; some observe closely their responses to weather or sun. Even if we don't consider ourselves to have 'communed' with plants, many of us who enjoy our gardens or houseplants have certainly listened to them on some level.

HISTORY OF HERBALS

Herbal lore was passed down orally for thousands of years before being written down. When European herbalists and botanists began writing books on plants and their medicinal uses – known as "herbals," books of recipes and cures for everyday ailments, offering a fascinating insight into healing of the time – they almost certainly would have sought knowledge from local folk healers for insights into the properties and uses of plants. The ancient knowledge passed down through these women was invaluable to these early academic botanists, herbalists and physicians (some acknowledged this, some didn't).

Some of the oldest surviving English herbal healing manuscripts are the Anglo-Saxon *Bald's Leechbook* and a medical compilation known as *Lacnunga,* both written about 900-950 CE and both of which live in the British Museum in London. In the *Leechbook* you'll find recipes for vapour and herb baths prescribed for all manner of ailments as well as 'smoke' for sick animals and humans with fragrant woods and dried herbs. When it comes to medicine and magic, the writings of our Anglo-Saxon ancestors provide a wealth of knowledge, rooted firmly in the land and Classical and European herbal traditions. These few surviving medical texts tell us of headache cures using betony, and herbs for improving digestion that are still used by some herbalists today, much as they were over a millennium ago.

The *Lacnunga* provides insight into early medieval theories of disease and healing. Of over a thousand herbal remedies within its pages, one of the best known is the "Nine Herbs Prayer" (sometimes called the "Nine Herbs

Charm"), which involves the preparation of nine plants as a treatment against poison and infection. (The numbers nine and three continue to be significant in paganism and various folklore.) The charm is sung three times over each of the herbs and to the patient. As Sheila Livingstone explains in her 1996 work, *Scottish Customs*, "To be really effective actions had to be accompanied by chants, often known only to a chosen few, especially seers and herb wives." This reflects a wisdom that it's not just the body that is part of the healing process: charms and incantations may help the mind and spirit too.

Now these nine herbs have power
against nine magic outcasts
against nine venoms
and against nine flying things.

Magical ideas are interwoven through these texts including prayers and invocations from both pagan and Christian origins: the "Nine Herbs Charm" refers to both Woden (Norse king of the gods, Odin) and Christ.

The Nine Herbs

In translations from Old English, the nine herbs of the charm are named as:

Mucgwyrt (mugwort)

Waybread (plantain)

Stune (watercress or Shepherd's Purse)

Stide (nettle)

Atterlothe (most commonly thought to be betony)

Maythen (camomile)

Wergulu (crab apple)

Fille & finule (chervil and fennel)

These herbs would be macerated together and made into a healing salve.

Mugwort *(Artemisia vulgaris)*, is a tall, feathery-leafed member of the daisy family that grows on wastelands. Mugwort is linked to the moon and magic, its Latin name comes from its association with the moon goddess, Artemis. Its common name is "mug weed" because it was used to flavour ale and beer before the use of hops.

It has antibacterial properties and can improve circulation. This was knowledge seemingly held by mermaids – an old Scottish myth tells of the "Mermaid of Clyde" (the river that runs through Glasgow and meets the sea at the Firth of Clyde) who mourned the death of a young woman of the city with a proverb of herbal recommendations:

> *If they wad drink nettles in March*
> *And eat muggins [mugwort] in May*
> *Sae many braw maidens*
> *Wadna go to clay.*[14]

Plantain, with its tough ribbed leaves and distinctive brown-centred cone-like flowers, was called "waybread" in ancient herbal texts for its propensity to grow along trails and roadside verges.

Jacob Grimm shared a tale about plantain. According to him, Plantain was once a maiden, who, worn out with constantly watching the roadway for her lover, was changed into a plant that still clings to a position by the wayside. In England, plantain has always had a high reputation as a healing herb and features in the works of both Chaucer and Shakespeare. Plantain was thought to draw out poisons, such as a poultice for a bee sting. It is still used today for insect bites and nettle stings. In the "Nine Herbs Charm," waybread has a particularly lovely verse dedicated to her:

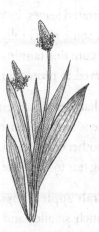

> *And you waybread*
> *plant mother*
> *eastward open*
> *within mighty*
> *over you chariots creaked*
> *over you queens rode*
> *over you brides trampled*
> *over you oxen snorted*
> *This all you then withstood*
> *and dashed apart*
> *as you withstand*
> *poison and infection*

and that evil
that fares through the land.

Watercress, so called because it grows in flowing streams, is a dark green leafy herb high in vitamin C. This peppery herb has been used both medicinally and as food for centuries, including in soup and tea. Victorians called it "Poor Man's Bread", as it was a need-food that could be easily foraged in times of famine. In the Old English of the "Nine Herbs Charm" this herb is called *Stune*; which has also been translated as Shepherd's Purse, another plant in the mustard family.

Nettle, with its stinging leaves, is mineral-rich, a restoring herb that relieves pain and reduces inflammation. Culpeper mentioned various nettles, describing their benefits thus: "Makes the heart merry, drives away melancholy, quickens the spirits…" He refers to them as "archangels," but also mentions that he expects this name was picked as a 'gloss' to make the common nettle sound more interesting! Here are words of the nettle from the charm:

Nettle she is called
stands she against poison
she drives out wretchedness
throws out poison.

Betony, once a common hedgerow plant, is now sadly quite rare due to changes in agricultural practices. With its purple trumpet-like flowers and serrated leaves, its value as a healing herb of medieval herbalists is reflected in some of its folk names including Heal-all, Self-heal, and Woundwort. It contains tannins that can help heal cuts and insect bites. It was also believed to protect one from witchcraft, as many herbs were thought to do.

Chamomile, a pretty white-petaled daisy-like flower with a distinctive grassy scent and fine leaves, reduces inflammation and helps wounds heal. It is a soother of nerves, skin and the digestive system. We still use it today for calming teas to settle the stomach and induce sleep and for gentle skin treatments.

Crab apple, *wergulu* in Old English, the wild apple of the hedgerows, much smaller and more sour than the cultivated apple, was a valuable source of vitamins and nutrients (and of course, cider).

Chervil and Fennel

Fille & finule
fela mihtigu twa þa wyrte.

"Chervil and fennel
very mighty these two plants."

Chervil, a relative of parsley, sometimes known as French parsley, is a calming and restorative herb and is used as a key ingredient in anti-wrinkle preparations marketed by major cosmetics companies today. Feathery-leafed fennel relieves nausea and reduces bleeding, it was also believed to impart strength and courage. Both herbs are calming and soothing, and are still used today with rich foods as a garnish. Some suggest that *fille* could also be thyme, a hardy, low-growing small-leafed herb with a strong flavour, which is known to have antiseptic properties, and so would also be a useful addition to this blend of herbs.

Many of the first printed texts in the English language were, similar to the *Lacnunga* and *Bald's Leechbook,* books about herbs and healing. We are lucky that we have access to any herbals from before the 1500s, as in England it was common for printed work on herbs, as well as topics such as astronomy and geography, to be destroyed because of their connection to magic, witches and occult arts and considered tainted with magic themselves.

The history of herbs is tightly woven through the work of healers and witches. It was common for superstition and magic to be involved in these texts in some way. In *Culpeper's Complete Herbal* – mistletoe, bay, betony and holly are all said to protect one from witchcraft. When Eleanour Sinclair Rohde wrote *The Old English Herbals* in 1922, she pointed out that writers of older herbals may well denounce witches and witchcraft as foolishness and superstitions, nevertheless, witches are still present in the folklore as well as a little of their magic in the herbal potions and charms. She says of yarrow, "one of the aboriginal English plants, and from time immemorial it has been used in incantations and by witches. Country folk still regard it as one of our most valuable herbs."

Monasteries were also a major source of herbal and medical knowledge in Europe and England during the early medieval period. Many Greek and Roman writings on medicine were preserved by the careful copying of manuscripts in monasteries, which had both the means and skill for writing. One such English monk, Bede, who I mention several times throughout this book, was an author of writings on English history, customs, and festivals. Bede created texts that are invaluable to our present-day knowledge of folklore and celebrations, particularly his work *De Temporum Ratione, (The Reckoning of Time)* in 725 CE.

Four Thieves

During an outbreak of the plague around 1772, four robbers plundered homes of ailing residents in Marseilles, France. But the thieves didn't fall sick themselves because they used a herbal tonic of vinegar. When caught, they agreed to share this protective recipe, which became known as Four Thieves Vinegar. And variations of this healing herbal mix have been created, shared and enjoyed by herbalists and wise women ever since. In more recent years, essential oil blends have been called Four Thieves Oil or Thieves Oil, even though these oil blends don't always have that much in common with the old vinegar recipe. (If you want to buy or to blend your own, look for sage or clary sage, angelica, clove, rosemary, marjoram and camphor.)

You will find many versions of this story and of the recipe; modern versions might include four herbs – one for each thief – to ward off cold and flu, much like the "Nine Herbs Charm" that protects from "nine flying things." Perhaps the "thieves" were actually ill health and infection, and these remedies protect one against that which could rob you of your health.

The chemist Rene Gattefosse, founder of modern aromatherapy, cites what he considers the original Four Thieves recipe in his 1937 book, *Gattefosse's Aromatherapy:*

Take three pints of strong white wine vinegar, add a handful of each of wormwood, meadowsweet, wild marjoram and sage, fifty cloves, two ounces of campanula roots, two ounces of angelic[a], rosemary and horehound and three large measures of camphor. Place the mixture in a container for fifteen days, strain and express, then bottle. Use by rubbing it on the hands, ears and temples from time to time when approaching a plague victim.

SPICE MAGIC

T he Kitchen Witch might gather herbs fresh from her garden or local woodland, but many other mainstays of magic, medicine and food-lore that are now part of our daily diets – spices, coffee and tea – come from further afield. Where herbs tend to refer to the soft leaves, flowers and roots of a plant, spices tend to be the harder and more aromatic parts which are always dried: berries, buds, bark, seeds and pods. In some cases, we get both a spice and herb from a plant, such as with the green fresh coriander and fennel and their useful dried seeds.

Exotic spices began to enter the British Isles when the Silk Road brought Asian spices and plants to Europe for the first time. Sea routes to India were discovered in the first century CE, and the Romans imported pepper, which spread throughout the empire, followed by the likes of nutmeg and cloves – for which they found tasty, medicinal, and to some, magical uses. Spices were also status symbols, precious jewels of the upper classes' dining rooms during the eleventh to thirteenth centuries. But slowly, slowly, they trickled down into the grasp of common folk. Culpeper's Complete Herbal (1653) refers to medicinal syrups made with cinnamon, nutmeg and ginger, and by the 1800s many people in Europe could afford these sweet and delicious exotic spices, and they started to appear in household cookery books.

Ayurveda

Each spice has a special day to it. For turmeric it is Sunday, when light drips fat and butter-colored into the bins to be soaked up glowing, when you pray to the nine planets for love and luck.

Turmeric which is also named halud, meaning yellow, colour of day-break and conch-shell sound. Turmeric the preservers, keeping foods safe in a land of heat and hunger. Turmeric the auspicious spice, placed on the heads of new-borns for luck, sprinkled over coconuts at pujas, rubbed into the borders of wedding saris.

Chitra Banerjee Divakaruni, *The Mistress of Spices* (1997)

The Mistress of Spices features women trained in India in the sacred art of herbs and spices, priestesses who revere the potential held within them. Though the story is fiction, it reflects many truths and ideas from Ayurveda about the value of spices and herbs.

The Indian practice of Ayurveda is many millenia old, a medical philosophy and practice that honours the power of plants. Translated as "knowledge of life," this ancient Indian holistic philosophy focuses on balancing mind, body and spirit.

At the heart of Ayurveda's teaching is a respect for nature and a humble appreciation for the magic of life. Ayurveda, in a way that witches may well recognise, sees our health in connection to everyone and everything around us: our family, our work, and our planet. Ayurvedic traditions use herbal wisdom and therapies to help treat and manage illness and chronic ailments, as well as illness prevention and vitality.

Cinnamon

The aromatic inner bark of the *Cinnamomum* tree, is warming and stimulating in scent and taste. In the laboratory of Louis Pasteur, the nineteenth century French bacteriologist, cinnamon was found to possess an antiseptic potential to destroy germs. Our ancestors rightly valued cinnamon as a preservative when they infused cinnamon with other spices in their mulled drinks; as well as a warming spice in cold months (now often saved for Christmas time).

Most cinnamon comes from trees grown in Sri Lanka, and when I visited Sri Lanka a few years ago whilst running an enchanting yoga retreat with my friend Trish, we watched men at a tea and spice plantation carefully peeling the curled bark of the cinnamon tree with sharp curved knives (while women outside picked the very top leaves of tea plants with delicate silver scissors).

Aniseed

Aromatic and liquorice-like in taste, aniseed is a member of the parsley family, and native of Egypt, but also extensively cultivated in Russia, Germany, and Spain. Comforting and soothing to the digestion, the medicinal virtues of aniseed are held in high esteem in Germanic traditions, and household bread was often flavoured with the whole seeds. *Bauernbrot,* "farmer's bread", is made with caraway, anise, and fennel seeds (all sweet, medicinal spices used to aid in digestion).

Star aniseed or star anise is from a different plant, the fruit of a small evergreen tree. Its name comes from the star-like form of the seed pod. The Japanese hold star anise in high regard, and it can be found planted near their temples; the seeds are burned as incense in sacred spaces.

Cardamom

Aromatic pods full of tiny black seeds, this spice is considered one of the oldest in the world in terms of its cultivation and use by humans. Many modern Kitchen Witches connect cardamom to Venus (goddess of love) and the element of water.

Cardamom originates from the Indian forests, and Ayurvedic medicine has used this spice to promote balance with warming properties that are soothing for the body. In fact, Indian Vedas (ancient texts) dating back over three thousand years ago attest to the digestive supporting properties of cardamom.

Cardamom, ginger and turmeric are in fact all members of the same botanical family: *Zingiberaceae.* And while very different plants, they do hold similar anti-inflammatory properties. In ancient Egypt, cardamom was used in cooking, medicine, perfumery, and Greeks and Romans also used it in their perfumes. Cardamom is added to coffee in Arabic, Bedouin, and Ethiopian cultures, in simple daily rituals of welcoming and hospitality that are still observed today. It is almost always included in Indian chai recipes for its aroma and warming, balancing qualities, as well as many sweet dishes. I think it is divine baked into bread and cakes.

Clove

Intense, aromatic, and spiky little devils when you're trying to push them into citrus fruits! Cloves are the dried flower buds of the clove tree with antimicrobial properties that are helpful in removing toxins. When applied externally in salves and balms they can offer pain relief from toothache, headache, and joint pain. The name "clove" derives from the Latin *clavus,* meaning nail. In Victorian England cloves were pushed into the skin of an orange to create a scented pomander, given as gifts and seen as a charm for good luck when gifted on New Year's Day. Nowadays they tend to be used as Christmas decorations.

Fennel

With a nutty, sweet flavour similar to liquorice or anise, the whole of the fennel plant can be eaten. Fennel bulbs are delicious roasted, stalks and feathery fronds can be used in salad, and dried fennel seeds make a sweet and soothing tea: fennel tea is popular today for digestion and is used for colic remedies for babies.

In Ayurveda herbal tea is prescribed to balance the doshas – the balance of elements within the body. Fennel tea is prescribed as cleansing and soothing. Other examples would be lemon tea to revitalise energy and flush out toxins and mint tea to clear one's head.

Common fennel *Foeniculum vulgare* was brought to Britain with the Romans and was made good use of by the Anglo-Saxons and was one of the herbs of the "Nine Herbs Charm," used to treat poison and infection.

In Greek Myth, Prometheus used a fennel stalk as a torch when he stole fire from the gods and gifted it to mortals on earth. In Roman myth, Silvanus, god of woods and forest, was sometimes crowned with fennel or depicted with a fennel stalk staff.

The word for fennel in ancient Greek is *marathon,* the city was named in honour of this place full of fennel plants. At the infamous Battle of Marathon, in those fennel fields, victory was claimed by the Greeks, and Athens' greatest runner, Pheidippides, became famous for running the 26 miles to Athens to announce the victory.

So, you can see perhaps where the superstitions that fennel supports fine athletes and victorious warriors may come from! Indeed, athletes, warriors, and later also Roman gladiators all ate fennel or rubbed themselves with fennel oil for success in battle and increased strength (as well as herbs such as mint, oregano and marjoram)…and victors were crowned with fennel foliage.

Ginger

Warming ginger root is used in Ayurveda to aid in many digestive problems. Chewing a small piece of ginger can soothe stomach aches, morning sickness and migraine. Having it as an infusion with lemon juice in warm water soothes the throat, alleviates nausea and helps treat the common cold. It is popular in many now classic European dishes where it was first used in its dried form in many cakes and biscuits, most famously, gingerbread. Its fresher counterpart arrived in the Middle Ages and was used in ginger ale and ginger wine. Young ginger roots are juicy and fleshy and can also be made into crystallised ginger sweets.

Nutmeg

The nutmeg tree, *Myristica fragrans* (meaning sweet-smelling), is a native of the Malay archipelago (a group of islands and countries also called the Spices Archipelago, which gives you a clue as to their major exports). Nutmeg is the seed of *Myristica fragrans*, from which we also get mace, the outer casing of the nutmeg. Sweet and musky, calming nutmeg can help ease you into a gentle sleep, which is why it is often added to warm milk sweetened with honey for a night-time drink. It is also served in comforting warm Christmas drinks like wassail, mulled wine and their German equivalent *gluhwein* (meaning *glow wine*). (See Section Four for a wealth of wisdom on the wassail and Yuletide beverages!)

Medieval Europeans first used it to flavour their beer. In the seventeenth and eighteenth centuries in Europe nutmeg was so popular that pocket-sized nutmeg graters were an indispensable accessory for men who would liberally season food, milky desserts, hot ale and punch with it.[*] And in modern Europe we still use nutmeg abundantly in our holiday baking – from German *Stollen* to British Christmas puddings and mince pies, to Norwegian *Julekak*. Like cinnamon, it is well connected to festivities and Yule in our minds, memories and kitchens.

> *Take some nutmeg and an equal weight of cinnamon and a bit of cloves, and pulverize them. Then make small cakes with this and fine whole wheat flower and water. Eat them often. It will calm bitterness of heart and mind, open your heart and impaired senses, and make your mind cheerful.*
> **Physica, Hildegard Von Bingen (1150). (Later translated from Latin by Priscilla Throop.)**

Pepper

Peppercorns are the dried berries of a flowering vine. Once the spice of royalty; they were placed in pharaohs' nostrils before burial. And like many spices were once very rare and expensive, used as both seasoning and medicine.

Now black pepper has become a main seasoning in Western cultures, and one of the most widely used spices worldwide. Added to most savoury dishes and sitting on the table next to the salt pot, we tend to forget about its medicinal qualities. It is known to be antibacterial in nature and was used to preserve food. In Ayurveda it is thought to increase internal heat, promote the free flow of oxygen to the brain, support digestion and circulation. And can be used to make a poultice used to draw out infection.

Pepper has been used in the past to refer to someone's or something's spirit and energy, and now we still refer to things that invigorate as having 'pep.' Pepper has no relationship with chilli and bell peppers, but chilli peppers are similarly boosters of heat.

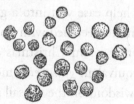

---

[*] But we should use it with caution, it can be toxic in large amounts, and servings of more than one teaspoon are not recommended.

Maternal Memory
– Khyati Patel

I was eighteen years old when I went back to India for the first time since moving to the UK aged seven. My Nani (maternal grandmother) and I took a trip to our ancestral village in Gujarat. She showed me how to cook my favourite meal of makai no rotolo and urad ni dhal, which is loosely translated as corn bread and split black gram dhal.

We went to the local flour grinder to buy locally-sourced corn flour, grown in a field two roads over. We collected cowpats, and she taught me how to pat them into patty cakes and throw them onto the wall so they would dry, ready to be used as fuel to cook our meal. It took forty-five minutes to get the fire going, requiring a lot of blowing into the smoke to ensure all parts of the cowpat were lit. Once lit, we were cooking. Just writing this, I can hear the birds outside on my Nani's veranda, as well as the strong smells of ghee and the spices being cooked for the dhal. I can see the skies above, expansive and lit by thousands of stars. We ate this meal with our hands. Together.

To me the memory is special because this artform of cooking no longer takes place, as most village homes have stoves, so reconnecting with nature on that level is lost. Cows are so sacred in India, so to use everything mother cow has to offer, and to not pollute nature by using gas is a wonderful way of reminding us that we belong to the earth. I really enjoy eating with my hands: it is the only way to eat Indian food. I love to have that sensory connection to food before you have even tasted, it is magical: to be enticed by the smells and visuals of the yellow hues of cornbread and dhal.

My family all eat this meal on most get-togethers during the cold winter months. Dhal and Rotolo is our winter bangers and mash: hearty, warming and if you give in to the pleasure of food, magical. That's the beauty about food, it connects all, and this meal is just that for me: a connection to my roots whilst living in the West.

MAGIC BEANS...COFFEE, CHOCOLATE...AND TEA

The Fables of the First Coffee

Coffee has had a rich history as it has travelled around the world, and there is a huge range of folktales and superstitions that feature coffee. Perhaps it is its long history of use as a tool for divination that has imbued it with a certain mystical quality: a connection to the otherworldly and the fantastic. Coffee can be an everyday magic.

One coffee origin story involves a Moroccan Sufi mystic. When travelling in Ethiopia, the legend goes, he observed birds of exceptional vitality feeding on berries and, upon trying the berries, experienced the same vitality.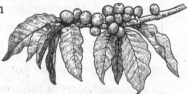

In another story, a disciple was once exiled from Mecca to a desert cave. Starving, he chewed berries from nearby shrubbery, but found they were bitter. He discovered, however, that roasting and boiling them resulted in a fragrant brown liquid which was revitalising and sustaining. His miracle discovery was held in great awe, and the disciple was allowed to return home and elevated to sainthood, whilst the coffee he discovered percolated throughout the world.

In another story, an Ethiopian goat-herder noticed the energising effects when his flock snacked on the bright red berries of a certain bush and tried the fruit himself. He brought the berries to a nearby monastery, but a monk, in disapproval, threw them into the fire. From that fire, an enticing aroma billowed as these berries roasted. The remaining beans were raked from the embers, ground up, and added to hot water, creating a beverage that kept one awake for hours – just the thing for those devoted to long hours of prayer.

Coffee, like the witches, has had its time of being condemned by the Church, which saw its effects as akin to alcohol and drugs. Some reacted to this beverage with suspicion and alarm. And, apparently, local clergy condemned coffee when it came to Venice in 1615 with intrepid European travellers from the mysterious and mystical lands of the East, as they were distrustful of this dark, exotic and intoxicating liquor.

I particularly enjoy the story that coffee controversy was so great that Pope Clement VIII was asked to assist. He decided to taste the beverage before making a judgment. Finding the drink satisfying, he gave it papal approval and then blessed coffee beans. With his blessing, coffee was free to be drunk by Catholics around the world. This story, like many legends, can't be authenticated, but it's still one of the more pleasant papal tales.

Despite the controversy, coffee houses quickly become centres of social activity in the major cities of England and through Europe in the 1600s. For the price of a cup of coffee, one could engage in stimulating conversation, games, and, perhaps most crucially, gossiping, arguing and discussing the breaking news of the day. These coffee houses soon became known as a place to catch up on news of the world and discuss ideas, creating a link between coffee and creative thought, ideas, inspiration, still very much alive today amongst artists, writers and business people as creative rocket fuel!

French historian Jules Michelet (who also wrote a very poetic book about witches: *La Sorcière* in 1862) saw coffee as "mighty nourishment of the brain, which unlike other spirits, heightens purity and lucidity; coffee, which clears the clouds of the imagination and their gloomy weight; which illuminates the reality of things suddenly with the flash of truth."

Coffee: The Liquid Ritual
– Mercedes Reyes, founder of the Bruja Coffee Co.

Coffee has always been a mystical brew, first consumed by humans in Ethiopia and spread into Yemen with the Sufi mystics. Coffee supported the evening devotional practice of rhythmic chants late into the night.

My own connection to coffee and its spirit is very intimate. I was born in Puerto Rico, and coffee was grown around me; it was roasted around me; it is part of the land I was born in. From a very early age, I saw the reverence in which coffee farmers and roasters treated the sacred plant. I was also taught to use it in ceremony and give it as an offering to gods and goddesses.

I learned to roast and make coffee with intention, from plant to cup. My way of roasting uses traditional firewood roasting practices. I use consecrated clay or cast-iron pots, and while roasting, instilling each batch of coffee with intention. I choose what moon phases to make certain roasts; it also helps that the coffee plants used for our coffee have been blessed. Intention and personal meaning are essential in ritual – sequences of actions we follow regularly, performed daily, fuelled by a powerful intention – separating it from everyday routine.

I consider coffee a magical libation and a gift from the Goddess. I am a Coffee Witch – a *bruja*[*] : I make coffee with intention and always will!

Black (Coffee) Magic

I drink coffee as part of my morning ritual, so I like to put in a little spice magic to start my day.

☾ Cinnamon – for prosperity.

☾ Cardamom – love, and to find flow in your day.

☾ Cloves – cleansing, ward against negative energies.

☾ Ginger – energising, invites success and motivation.

☾ Salt – cleansing, dispels negativity.

Other ideas:

☾ Place intent into your morning coffee by meditating on what the day holds for you as it brews and think about what you want from the day before you.

☾ Stirring your brew clockwise can invite positivity and growth, and anti-clockwise reduces, banishes, or casts away the undesired.

☾ Brew yourself a cup of coffee and try scrying. In a dark, quiet room light some candles. Gaze into your coffee, your 'black mirror,' and let your mind wander. Consider the darkness of the coffee and think about the dark, rich aspects of your own life. What parts of your life

---

* *Brujería* is a Spanish word for witchcraft. *Brujas* are healers, intuitive advisers and workers of magic. *Brujería* has roots in several spiritual lineages, and it can refer to various spiritual practices from African, Caribbean, and indigenous Latin American peoples. Like the word witch, it can bring out powerful reactions in people and is not always used positively, but many are taking steps to reclaim these words of magic and power, and their place in the modern world.

need stimulating? What aspects of the darkness do you enjoy? When you have explored the questions, you can close the practice by drinking your magical brew.

(Leave a cup of coffee out overnight on a table or the kitchen counter, along with a slice of bread to help keep away ghosts or to appease mischievous spirits.

(Finally, I enjoy a cup with my morning yoga practice, savouring the aroma and warmth; it helps me focus, find my grounding and fills me with gratitude.

A few more ideas from Sarah:

(As you start your morning or take a pause from your busy day for a cup, bring your attention to its warmth, scent and taste. Maybe you connect those coffee grounds with grounding and mental clarity or with energising and speeding up. Maybe your morning cup is your morning ritual, a peaceful treat: hands warmed around this simple potion. Maybe you use this time to ponder the future or simply enjoy the here and now.

CHOCOLATE

Ah, precious chocolate! Even with no knowledge of its origins, many of us would agree it is special and sacred! The Latin name of the cacao plant *Theobroma cacao*, means "food of the gods" (*Theos:* gods and *broma:* food). This would not have been its original name, originating in Central America as it does. As always with the origins of words, there is hot debate on this. Etymologists trace the origin of the word "chocolate" to the Mesoamerican[†] words such as *xocoatl/chicolatl/cacahuatl*, which may refer to drinks brewed from cacao[‡] beans.

---

† Mesoamerica is a historical region and cultural area that extends through Mexico, Guatemala, and Costa Rica, and where cultures such as Aztecs, Mayan and Olmec originated.
‡ Cacao refers to the raw, unroasted beans, whereas cocoa refers to the beans once roasted and ground, as usually used in Western confectionary.

The Cacao Pharmacy

Theobromine: a compound obtained from cacao seeds. It is an alkaloid resembling caffeine in its effects to awaken and enliven. You can harness its powers if you sprinkle cacao nibs on your morning oatmeal.

Magnesium: an essential mineral for the human body, helping with muscle and nerve function, regulating blood pressure, and supporting the immune system. Cacao along with almonds and cashew nuts, are right at the top of the list of foods highest in magnesium. So, chocolate bars with high cocoa content (like dark chocolate) are also very high in magnesium. Some studies have found that taking magnesium supplements could help soothe PMS symptoms, such as mood swings and bloating. (Something many women have known intuitively for a long time!)

Cacao also has **anti-inflammatory and antioxidant** properties that may have a positive influence on immune health. **Tryptophan**, found in raw, unprocessed cacao, helps our bodies produce serotonin, the neurotransmitter which can support mood, digestion, sleep, memory. You can see how the power of cacao helped it become a ceremonial and healing drink.

The ancient civilisations like the Olmec, Mayans and Aztecs all celebrated the powers of cacao. Mayans saw chocolate as the drink of the gods, brewing roasted and ground cacao seeds mixed with chillies, honey and spices, pouring the liquid from one pot to another, creating a thick foamy draught. The Mayan goddess of cacao, IxCacao (literally Cacao Woman) was earth goddess and mother of the abundance of cacao and all foods. During menopause and childbirth, women drank chocolate to fortify themselves.[15]

Carvings and decorations suggest that Aztec dignitaries consumed chocolate as an offering to the great god of the forest, Quetzalcoatl, as well as the goddess of fertility, Xochiquetzal, and that cacao was hugely valuable and used as currency.

Expeditions in the 1500s brought cacao to Europe and the wider world. Chocolate (a distortion of some of the suggested roots of the original Mesoamerican names) was often mixed with sugar, honey, vanilla and cinnamon and it quickly became popular among the wealthy who could afford it and the sweeteners it needed. When it reached the British Isles, special "chocolate houses" appeared even earlier than the popular coffee houses I mentioned earlier. As the trend spread, many nations set up cacao plantations in countries along the equator.

In the present day you may have seen cacao ceremonies offered as spiritual rituals, workshops and at retreats and festivals. They are very popular, but this is no 'new age' idea. Like many of the best ideas, it is ancient and sacred in its origins. Luxurious cacao mixed with the likes of cinnamon, cardamom and anise seeds brewed and consumed with reverence. With this magic of intention, of creating something with care and love cacao has, for some, come full circle. Journeying from the sacred medicine of nobility to sumptuous treat and everyday snack, and for some, back to the sacred in ceremony once again.

Its magical powers and ability to enchant are celebrated in many fictional works including Laura Esquivel's *Like Water for Chocolate* and Joanne Harris' *Chocolat* – to name a couple of my personal favourites – where women (like Tita and Vianne) weave magic and love into their cacao creations and respect the power of the food they prepare. And some special women are bringing back these ancient magical practices too. Moontime Chocolate in Devon, UK combines healing herbs, fruit and nuts with raw cacao to support women's bodies and minds throughout the menstrual cycle. And the Bruja Coffee Co. based in America, builds on long traditions with ceremonial cacao elixirs made with cacao beans and cinnamon from Oaxaca and cacao beans from Guatemala and Puerto Rico.[16]

A Story of Chocolate Witches

By the time chocolate was making its way into Europe, Latin American women were brewing it daily in their homes. Cacao's long history of ritual and curative properties would have been passed down through recipes and generations. And just as in Britain at this time one may have consulted a cunning woman, in Latin America, one may consult a *hechizera* (sorceress) or *bruja* (witch) and everyone, from slaves to nobility, sought potent potions and magical incantations for revenge, escape, resolution, to entice lovers and spurn enemies. When the

Inquisition[*] swept through Latin America, they sought to persecute these chocolate-brewing witches.

During the Inquisition many women were imprisoned and tortured on charges of (amongst other things) witchcraft, heresy and using folk practices. Many were specifically accused of practising magic through bewitched chocolate. Professor Martha Few spotted this trend from the remaining Inquisition archives, and it is from her work, as a trailblazer in this field, that I mainly draw from here.[17]

In the Inquisition testimonies, Professor Few found chocolate appeared with some frequency, many cases centred around the potent chocolate concoctions created by women to carry potions and poisons, that might be infused with herbs, powders, and bodily fluids and hairs.

Professor Few reveals some inspiring stories from Guatemala, such as churchmen becoming enraged by women who would, with their maids, consume steaming mugs of hot chocolate in church, disrupting services in little chocolate rebellions.[†] And one woman who had a quarrelsome reputation was named by locals *La Panecito* (the pastry) because of a rumour that she killed a woman by poisoning her with "bewitched chocolate pastries." And at least one husband was so afeared his wife would bewitch his morning hot chocolate that he reported in records that he was forced into the 'unnatural' act of actually making it for himself and serving a cup to her too (gasp!).

Members of the Inquisition, like the witch hunters of Europe, saw a powerful woman as scary, but a powerful group of women…terrifying. And the practice of magic and folk healing often brought women together, seeking cures and potions from indigenous healers and wise women.

Authorities and civilians increasingly associated chocolate with not

* The Inquisition was set up by the Catholic Church to uncover and punish heresy throughout Europe and the Americas. It began in the 1200s, with the pope appointing the first inquisitors, and continued for hundreds of years. Targets included heretics, healers, witches, Protestants, people of different religions and those who held superstitions or folk beliefs. When the Spanish Inquisition moved through Mexico and into South America in the 1570s, people were imprisoned, tortured, and burned alive.

† The collective noun for solid chocolate is, as far as I can tell, a bar or box. But I think "a rebellion of chocolate" sounds very fine indeed!

only magic, but also a rebellion and empowerment that could cut across racial and status boundaries. Mixed-race, indigenous and African wise women, healers, and midwives all might mingle in markets and kitchens and at births and sickbeds, sharing practices from different cultures and countries, for homemade cures and crafts that bordered somewhere between science and magic. Women's connections to ritual, cooking, healing, and ancient religions were part of their cultural authority and power. And chocolate was a bewitching symbol of that held power.

TEA AND SYMPATHY

Tea, although not a native plant to the British Isles (it originates from Asia), has become a fundamental part of our culture here. Tea, coffee and chocolate all arrived in the British Isles around the 1600s. And each became popular with certain groups in society. At first, tea was a treat for nobility who could afford the sugar and sweet treats that turned 'taking tea' into a real occasion. At that time coffee was the cheaper beverage. But as prices dropped with trading deals and colonialism tea was, by 1800, consumed by virtually everyone, from royalty to factory worker to farmer. And it continues to be popular today and available to all, and is pretty much considered a cure for everything, from broken hearts to a shock, to offer visitors with biscuits, a morning staple and afternoon refreshment.

In England there are cream teas (a pot of tea accompanied by scones, cream, and jam), afternoon tea (with sandwiches and dainty cakes to tide one over until evening meals), tea-time (another name for supper or dinner), not to mention the tea dance, tea party, tea breaks, oh, and elevenses (when one stops for a short break at 11, often for a cup of tea and a biscuit…or maybe a toasted tea cake). To offer 'tea and sympathy' is to offer care, a kindly ear, and a 'cuppa' to someone who is upset. I could write a whole chapter here about the power of a nice cup of tea. But this quote, somehow, to me, just says it perfectly:

The true spiritual home of the teapot is surely in a softly-lighted room, between a deep armchair and a sofa, two cups only, awaiting their fragrant infusion, whilst the clock points nearer to six than five, and a wood fire flickers sympathetically on the hearth.

Agnes Jekyll, "Kitchen Essays" (1922)

This is the simple, beautiful, magic that can be found at the hearth and within a warm cup.

Tasseomancy

Tasseomancy is a form of divination that interprets patterns in tea leaves, coffee grounds, or wine sediments. In fact, anything can be used for divination as humans have sought to interpret what the threads of life may have in store for them. In ancient Egypt and Mesopotamia, oil and inks were added to bowls of water. Towards the end of the medieval period in Europe, fortune-tellers might use tarot cards (the first decks appeared in Italy around 1440), but many could give 'readings' from drink sediment, splatters of wax, or the way items like stones and bones fell.

Reading Tea Leaves by "a Highland Seer," written in the eighteenth century, is thought to be the oldest book on tasseomancy in English (although the practice is many centuries older). Offering sets of symbols to interpret tea-leaf patterns, the book talks of Scottish "spae wives" (from the Norse spa, meaning prophecy) regarding their teacups to tell of things to come.

Tea-leaf readers might also call door-to-door to offer their services, and it became quite a popular entertainment during the upsurge in the popularity of spiritualism in the Victorian era. Ladies might host social gatherings that centred around tea and divining, and potteries made fortune telling cups to keep up with demand, printed with images such as zodiac symbols. Practice varies through cultures, but some images are universal: if within the grounds, you see symbols of hearts, coins, or flowers, you may expect to find connections to love and prosperity.

SECTION THREE SUMMARY

As modern medical advances occurred, using herbs was cast as archaic. A remnant of the superstitious past, it was demonised via connections to the wise ones that still used them. Both the cunning women and their herbs became less trusted and more feared. Luckily for us, some of the knowledge was passed down through families and communities as folk medicine and healing practices. Almost all of us will recall a remedy their grandmother used to make, or a superstition involving ritual, like leaving a cake out for the fae folk, rubbing nettle stings with dock leaves or throwing salt over one's shoulder. While many cultures never really lost touch with their herbal practices, like Indian Ayurveda and Chinese herbal medicine, Western practices have become something of an amalgamation of fragments of traditions, as they had to be passed down in whispers for generations.

Medical science is beginning to find value in some of this ancient plant knowledge, and research into traditional uses and benefits of herbs for such major health issues as malaria have yielded amazing results.[*]

Pharmacists in the West now know that plants like chamomile and lavender are soothing to the body because they contain chemicals that can have a sedative effect on the nervous system. In many different peer-reviewed clinical trials on lavender essential oil[18] it has been shown to be as effective as branded sedatives and antidepressants in many people and to treat issues such as migraines. This might not be suitable for everyone, but it is exciting nonetheless, as lavender has far fewer side effects than many pharmaceutical drugs and can be grown yourself, which is no small thing in places where drugs are not affordable or easily accessible.

The Saxon healer would have known the spirit of both chamomile and lavender comforts the mind and relaxes the body and can promote healing. It's not that one way is right and one wrong, but we have different ways of viewing the body and understanding healing. Just as the Chinese medicine system sees meridian lines, yogis see chakras, Saxons saw spirits of plants that

---

[*] A great example is sweet wormwood *(Artemesia annua)* mentioned in a fourth century Jin dynasty text, for treating the malaria symptom of fever. Scientist Tu Youyou won the Nobel Prize in 2015 for her work in which she isolated the artemisinin compound in sweet wormwood and created a drug that has made a huge difference in the management of malaria treatment in the world.

could soothe and nourish the spirit in the body.

In the past a vast realm of what we would consider complementary and alternative health and healing modalities today would have fallen under the broad umbrella of cunning folk and folk magic: homoeopaths, counsellors, aromatherapists, herbalists, hypnotherapists, mediums, clairvoyants and spiritual healers. We may not call them cunning folk and wise ones anymore, but they are still with us (to our great benefit). So can we look back and really pay attention to what the women and wise ones were saying (and what their counterpart say now)? Can we look at the craft of the herb wives, alewives, herbalists, and learn from it? Can we do our best to see and hear the witches, the women and men, behind the rituals and superstitions? Can we learn, again, to see the magic and medicine in what we eat? I hope so.

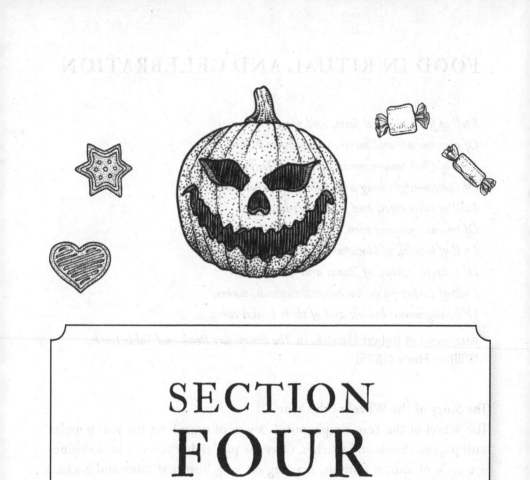

SECTION
FOUR

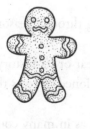

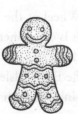

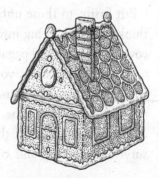

FOOD IN RITUAL AND CELEBRATION

I tell of festivals, and fairs, and plays,
Of merriment, and mirth, and bonfire blaze;
I tell of Christmas-mummings, New Year's day,
Of twelfth-night king and queen, and children's play
I tell of valentines, and true-love's-knots,
Of omens, cunning men, and drawing lots:
I tell of brooks, of blossoms, birds, and bowers,
Of April, May, of June, and July flowers
I tell of May-poles, hock-carts, wassails, wakes,
Of bridegrooms, brides, and of their bridal cakes.

Attributed to Robert Herrick, in *The Every-day Book and Table Book*,
William Hone (1826)

The Story of the Wheel of the Year

The Wheel of the Year, simply put, is a way of organising the year popular
with pagans, druids and witches. Over the past eighty years or so, a distinctive cycle of annual festivals, drawing on long historical roots and ancient
celebrations, have been grouped together in a modern framework. The Wheel
of the Year, also called The Witches' Year, is both old and new; echoes of
many pre-Christian and pagan practices can be seen within its many variations, along with once common folk-festivals. Agricultural points of the year
are planted in between observable solar events of equinoxes and solstices, in
whose honour many Neolithic stone circles were made.

This is the template I'll use to outline food and feasting through seasonal
rituals and celebrations.

But firstly, to those unfamiliar with the Wheel of the Year or its history, I
think it's worth going into briefly here, as it is often mentioned in texts that
cover witchcraft and paganism, mine included.

Here's how it began, you might say. In the British Isles, as in many countries, we began as hunter-gatherers: people in tune with the earth, stars, seasons, who would, in time, create settlements, cultivate crops, and domesticate
animals. Knowledge of the weather and seasons was the foundation of our
survival: watching and celebrating the sun's set and rise; snows and frosts

melting; green shoots appearing; animals giving birth and giving milk; crops ripening. Traditions, rituals and offerings grew up around these celestial, agricultural and seasonal cycles. They became special and sacred occasions, marked by the ritual preparation and consumption of food. To come together in feasts is part of our very earliest communal acts, from the dawn of human society. Festivals were feast times and a much-anticipated break from what may have been a frugal and monotonous diet in rural communities.

Winter
Solstice

Samhain

Imbolc

Autumn
Equinox

Spring
Equinox

Lughnasadh

Beltaine

Summer
Solstice

Whilst these celebrations of gratitude brought the whole community together to eat, drink and make merry, they were also a time of fear and reverence; sacrifices and offerings were made to deities to seek protection in the dark and cold seasons that could well claim lives and crops. Appeals may have been made for the return of the sun at a time when no one could know for sure that it would. And in some ways, we see this fear embodied at festival times in forms such as folkloric tales of malevolent beings, ghosts, spirits, and fearsome seasonal monsters cast into the world at these special threshold points.

Ancient Calendar Forms

Celtic cultures had perhaps the biggest influence on the modern Wheel of the Year as it sought to draw from (but was not limited to) the native customs of the British Isles. We have limited physical calendars that remain from the ancient Celtic world. The Gaulish Coligny calendar is the oldest known example, dating from the second century. It's not a wheel but a tablet, and we have just fragments of it, and it features only the faintest echoes of what has been drawn forward into modern-day observance. Like the month named *Samoni/ Samonios* is thought to be related to the word Samhain – as summer's end.

Other calendrical devices that have survived are much larger in size. Ancient stone monuments were used to track the position of the sun and align with equinoxes and solstices. Some of the most well-known of these ancient calendrical structures are Stonehenge in England, Newgrange in Ireland and Maeshowe in the Orkney Islands. They are believed to be upwards of 3000 years old and are all perfectly aligned in some way to the solstice sun's rising and setting. For Newgrange and Maeshowe, their central chambers are illuminated on the Winter Solstice, at Stonehenge, the setting sun once shone through the largest trilithon (stone arch) – and would today, if it was still standing. Other stones line up with sunrise on Summer Solstice.

Sometimes the most powerful magic is the simplest; as simple as a rising and setting sun. The sun, its power and its cycles are central to our survival as a species and the growing of food. It is no wonder that it has been so carefully observed, celebrated and formed a central part of most religious and magical traditions.

A circle is perhaps the oldest symbol of the sun, and circles containing crosses were used to symbolize the sun and its journey through the year and seasons. Sun wheels and solar crosses are another calendrical form, again, with shadows of our modern Wheel of the Year. The eight-spoked wheel icon appears widely though ancient cultures from the Dharma wheel in Hindu and Buddhist cultures, to Ancient Greek and Norse runic symbols. The sun was both a symbol and a very real source of strength, energy and life itself, and though cultures' meanings may have varied, striking similarities exist. In Europe such icons were offered at shrines, in carvings, worn as amulets, cast into coin form, thrown into rivers and buried in tombs from at least

Palaeolithic times. Some had four spokes,* Celtic wheels might have six or eight spokes. And Wheels featuring six and eight spokes can be found on the imagery on the Gundestrup cauldron (a stunning artefact of European Iron Age silver work). Sun wheels resembled chariot wheels and were almost certainly connected in imagery, joined in their symbolic turning. For the Greeks, Apollo was believed to carry the sun across the sky each day in his chariot. For the Celts, the sky god Taranis was often depicted with a lightning bolt in his right hand, and a sun wheel in his left.

Following the Wheel to the Witch

Easter-fires, magdag-fires, midsummer-fires with their numerous ceremonies, carry us back to heathen sacrifices; especially such customs as rubbing the sacred flame, running through the glowing embers, throwing flowers into the fire, baking and distributing large loaves or cakes, and the circular dance.
Jacob Grimm, *Deutsche Mythologie* (1835)

The Wheel of the Year is now primarily celebrated by witches and pagans interested in reclaiming pre-Christian celebrations. It marks the basic seasons of the year according to the movements of the sun and the earth. These important way-markers of the year in the British Isles since the Middle Ages, include not only when seeds were sown and harvests gathered, but dates when rents were due, school terms started and by which debts and disagreements had to be legally settled. These dates were followed by everyone, for thousands of years; it was only into the modern era, that they became more closely connected to witches...

Folk traditions and superstition never forgot how figures like the witches and the older pagan holidays were connected, in ways good and bad. Some especially feared witches at this time, others thought that as townsfolk gathered to celebrate their festivals, the witches also held their own special ceremonies. The idea that witches travel to meetings of other witches and otherworldly beings, featured heavily in early modern texts and trial records, creating a body of folklore and superstition. There were many stories of witches in-

---

* The four-spoked wheel could connect to the seasonal wheel known to almost all in the western world: the cycle of spring, summer, autumn and winter. This is an even simpler circular way of viewing the year that you may prefer.

verting popular festivals, turning the good into bad: the festivals becoming diabolical, the Mass becoming a demonic "Black Mass" were part of an idea that these people were mocking or destroying the customs of the Church, creating merriment and mischief in settings outside the Church. This, alongside their supposed dealings with the Devil made them heretics in the eyes of both Church and lawmakers – rejecting religion and, as such, the monarchy.

Tales of the Witches' Sabbaths to which they flew on their broomsticks to dance with the Devil, and cast malefic magic represented a flipping of what was portrayed as the social norms: being obedient, restrained and going to church to observe Christian festivals. A key part of the issue here was that these stories represented a mockery of the Church, which they were not happy about (to put it mildly).

The idea of the Witches' Sabbath was a huge part of the witch hunts and witch trials, even though it was essentially fiction. But if there were no real Witches' Sabbaths and Black Masses, why did people take this fantasy so seriously? Perhaps, like the best tales, the stories were based around *some* facts and real events: celebrations and dancing at key dates, but also sickness, ships sinking in winter storms, hopes and fears of food and hunger, festivals of lighting fires and a little intoxication, on dates that were followed by most communities, all these things really did happen. Just as there existed women who could help heal a burn with herbs or had a knack of predicting the future. The dark fantasies of the witch hunters were just that: fantasy. But ideas of great secret organisations and vast cults of witches remained popular...

The Witch-Cult Idea

The other rites – the feasts and dances – show that it was a joyous religion; and as such it must have been quite incomprehensible to the gloomy Inquisitors and Reformers who suppressed it.

Margaret Murray, *The Witch-Cult in Western Europe* (1921)

Scholars, writers and historians created works from 1800s onwards through which they shared more about the festivals, deities and ceremonies involved in rural customs to a far wider audience during a revival of interest in folklore.

And many picked up on these ideas like Jules Michelet (who wrote *La Sorciere* in 1862), George James Frazer (*The Golden Bough*, 1890), Robert Graves (*The White Goddess*, 1948) Margaret Murray (see above) and Gerald Gardner, founder of Wicca. All these authors played with the idea – with varying levels of historical fact and fictional imagination – that the witches of history had followed pre-Christian pagan religions and ancient observances based on the agricultural cycle, craft and tradition in their gatherings. Many of the books were intrigued by an idea of one great religion of witches spanning Europe and the world (I imagine what tied them together was probably more primal and intuitive than religion) and explored ideas of ancient goddess cults, the festivals, deities, and ceremonies. Work like this inspired, and continues to inspire, writers and thinkers to explore the lives, practices and contributions of witches and women.

Margaret Murray, in her book *The Witch-Cult* in Western Europe (1921), used the testimonies of the accused witches, and built on this idea of festivals and their importance specifically to the witch. I should say from the outset that her work is "dismissed and discredited"[*] by many peers and scholars for basing many of her theories on scant evidence – something that is often exhaustively stated when referring to her work (so much so that I was loathe to mention it, after all there are inaccuracies and wild statements in many books of witchcraft and Wicca – but perhaps Murray's position and influence in academia made her subject to harsher criticism).

Murray tried to listen for the voices, however faint, of the persecuted and using what records remained from witch trials, as well as folklore surrounding European witchcraft and made an attempt to create a structure around the ritual gatherings, which would provide the blueprint for the contemporary religion of Wicca. (Gerald Gardner and Murray were friends and her books feature testimonies from accused witches that touch on ideas on covens, sabbaths, books and festivals which would later show up in Gardner's work.)

The festival days, as Murray identifies them in her book, are:

> *The four actual days are given in only one trial, that of Issobell Smyth at Forfar in 1661, 'By these meitings shee mett with him [the Devil] every quarter at Candlemas, Rud-day,[†] Lambemas, and Hallomas.'*

---

[*]   Just to give you an idea, an article by Jacqueline Simpson in *Folklore,* the journal of The Folklore Society in 2012 starts with this paragraph:
"No British folklorist can remember Dr Margaret Murray without embarrassment and a sense of paradox. She is one of the few folklorists whose name became widely known to the public, but among scholars her reputation was deservedly low; her theory that witches were members of a huge secret society preserving a prehistoric fertility cult through the centuries is now seen to be based on deeply flawed methods and illogical arguments."
[†]   In Scotland Rud-day was connected to May Day/Beltane.

Murray also notes other notable dates mentioned, predominately Christian festivals:

Both generations of Lancashire witches (1613 and 1633) kept Good Friday. Jonet Watson of Dalkeith (1661) was at a meeting 'about the tyme of the last Baille-ffyre night'. The Crook of Devon witches (1662) met on St. Andrew's Day, at Yule. In Connecticut (1662) the 'high frolic' was to be held at Christmas.

All of these festivals mentioned were very common, enjoyed by the majority of folks in the British Isles and Europe, including the accused witches. To many looking back now, we can see that these were the festivals of 'ordinary folk' that kept coming up in testimonies, which is very telling of the folk who were being accused of witchcraft: they were ordinary people too.

Some witches may have had a little more awareness of the ancient pagan practices that inspired the festivities, maybe with some workings or charms on auspicious dates, their celebration may have looked a little different from, say, the local church services. But most people in the British Isles would have celebrated some or all of the festivals in the Wheel of the Year in some manner.

So, as we look at the dates noted on the Wheel of the Year, it's important to note that these were never festivals that were celebrated only by witches, and the same is true today. These were and are dates celebrated by many from pagan to farmer, from churchgoer to anyone with Celtic family history. The land was (and is) the true calendar of witches and non-witches alike, and certainly in modern day the Wheel is useful to and used by many.

Wicca and the Wheel

In the 1950s, Gerald Gardner self-identified as a witch and began the process of founding Wicca as a religion with help from notable witches such as Doreen Valiente. Texts, poems and folklore were drawn on and the first Wiccan seasonal rites and invocations were created. By the late 1950s, Wiccan and druid groups had adopted eightfold ritual calendars, a neat cycle with a celebration and opportunity to meet and feast every six weeks or so. And the Wheel of the Year became the yearly cycle of witches' holidays for practitioners of the religion of Wicca, but the holidays and structure were also adopted by many solitary witches and pagans too.

The Celtic people of Britain and Ireland called Candlemas Imbolc or Oimelc, May Eve Beltane, Lammas Lughnassadh, and Hallowe'en Samhain. These were the four great festivals of the pagan year, and are frequently referred to in Celtic mythology.

Doreen Valiente, *Witchcraft for Tomorrow* (1978)

In *Witchcraft for Tomorrow,* Valiente names the four festivals, along with the solstices and equinoxes she called the 'Sabbats.' Other Wiccan groups in 1970s would assign names to the Summer Solstice: Litha – an Anglo-Saxon word referring to gentle season of summer. Yule was brought in from Germanic customs, but was already in more common usage mentioned by Frazer, Valiente, Gardner and Murray in their books, and equinox holidays were given other names (Ostara and Mabon). These names gradually grew in popularity.

Gardner, Murray and Valiente, for all the flaws one may see in some of their ideas of ancient lineage, succeeded in drawing out positive elements from a challenging history, (re)claiming the word 'witch', that had been pushed upon many people of the past. Wicca took disparate ideas, beliefs and practices and brought them together within a framework.

And frameworks like the Wheel of the Year, paired with the work of Wiccans, druids and pagans in the modern era, have helped to remind us how to bring some elements of food and celebrations back to the fore. Books from the 1990s like *A Kitchen Witch's Cookbook* by Patricia Telesco, *Magic in Food* by Scott Cunningham, and books of pagan homemaking by Dan and Pauline Campanelli, were fundamental in naming and laying out the path of the Kitchen Witch as we recognise it today. Authors such as these reconnected certain foods with festivals, but also helped magic become, once more, a part of everyday life for many.

Wheel of the Year – Past, Present, Future

Many of the older traditions of festivals – lighting fires, rituals for good luck, charms and offerings, celebrating the earth's cycles – are perfectly in line with what many see as the true nature of the witch, honouring and listening to the natural world. This is perhaps why those who identify with witchcraft and paganism have held onto rural traditions long after many folks moved to the cities and forgot about celebrating the harvest and other such traditions.

A journey through the Wheel of the Year is an exploration of how the

Kitchen Witches of old may have foraged the hedgerows, what superstitions and celebrations may have existed in their communities, what charms would have been cast, what ancient stories may have been told around the festival fires and what delicious foods were eaten. These celebrations can help us to connect to memory, traditions and reclaim some practices of past generations. The folklore of these long-intertwined festivals, customs and foods can guide us through the seasons today, just as much as in days gone by.

The superstitions, feasts and hearth crafts involved in these celebrations hold a special place in many generations' hearts and memories: the soul cakes, the figgy pudding, the cracking of nuts on the fire to seek hope and insight. These festivals, now so beloved of pagans, witches, and druids, are the celebrations of older communities and times. This is not just the witch's year, but it is the year of the Earth and our ancestors: all of us. These rituals give a sense of culture and history within a community, creating a shape and meaning to life throughout the year. As a species, we bond over shared practices, and the sharing of food is a strong example of this. Through these celebrations we also show gratitude and give something back to the unseen, which in turn strengthens the bonds between humans and what has been understood as the divine/otherworld/magic.

Some folk customs, such as balefires and blessing fields, are distinctly rural, whereas others might have been more popular in towns and cities. But much of the magic of these festivals starts in the kitchen – both urban and rural – with women, who before each of these festivals would be found making preparations: baking seasonal cakes, breads and feast dishes, brewing, decorating, making offerings of food, drink and prayer, following rituals and offering food on altars…doing the magic that women have practised for thousands of years.

For us today, food may have lost its value as a token of sacrifice and symbolic communication with deities, with the fairies, and with ancestors. Eating in season, calendars of feasting and fasting, distinctions between holiday and workday eating have perhaps blurred – especially for those living in cities and shopping from large supermarkets. But nothing is yet lost, we can still learn to do these things if we so wish. In these customs, we can hear the voices of people of the past. And we can bring their wisdom into the present, through the food we can all make and share.

JOURNEYING THE WHEEL OF THE YEAR

S o now we have explored the history of the Wheel, I will guide us through just some of the food, folklore and fairy tales of the seasons. It's important to stress before we dive in, that the Wheel of the Year is an attempt to draw many practices together. It's a lot to compress down into just eight festivals!

All the festivals of the year tend to be marked by fires and feasting, but each also has its own unique traditions reflecting the seasonal abundance of each region. Dates can vary with harvest, geographical, seasonal and astrological considerations.

I am aware that some may feel that their festivals have been left off, or have different names, or even that their festivals have been appropriated by putting them side by side with others. So if it all gets too exhausting or confusing, feel free to go outside, lay down on the grass and watch the trees: they'll tell you just fine what season it is and when it's changing...and you can mark it as you see fit.

For each festival we will cover:

(The background of the festival and varied names.

(Some of the folklore, themes and superstition surrounding the festivals.

(Food from the British Isles and other European countries connected with the festival.

(What is to be found in the hedgerow, farm, allotment, and garden at this time of year, or what to look out for in the shops and farmers' market.

(Celebratory food ideas and activities as we further explore how to bring ancient and modern practices together and celebrate in the present day.

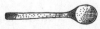

SAMHAIN

The thinning veil is our curtain up, our doorway, our threshold into the journey around the Wheel of the Year.

Many modern witches and pagans have adopted Samhain as their year-end, so to many, this is New Year's Eve. There are various theories as to when the calendar year begins in ancient pagan and Celtic schedules. Celtic folk scholars John Rhys and James George Frazer suggested a Samhain end/start to the year, which is still a popular idea with many neo-pagans and Celtic traditions. Samhain marks the end of the harvest period and the start of winter. All is gathered and drawn in as summer comes to a close. It is a time for endings, before the dormancy of winter and rebirth in spring. People may have viewed this time as the death of the year, which it was, in many ways.

This seasonal transition from late autumn into winter would be special and significant in all ancient farming cultures. The end of October and into November in the northern hemisphere[*] was when all of the manual field labour was completed, the harvest reaped and valuable foodstuffs preserved. People would finally have a chance to slow down from a busy and challenging pace of life ready for the dark months ahead.

Samhain is one of the four fire festivals, marked by bonfires or balefires (names drawn from burning bones and/or bales of hay) symbolised light, order and protection in the darkness. Sometimes the ashes were used to bless both people and livestock. Household fires would be extinguished and re-lit from the communal Samhain fire, a practice that dates back at least to ancient Greece and Rome, when homes would light their hearth from the communal temple fire for goddess Hestia/Vesta.

In many cultures, this time of year became a chance to reflect on the dear departed, to visit cemeteries and tend graves. Families would gather for special dinners where they would share memories and stories of their beloved ones and ancestors.

Some of the earliest details of Samhain, as we know it today, come from medieval Celtic records. Along with feasting and celebration, it has a reputation as when "the veil" between the living and the dead was at its thinnest, in con-

---

[*] In Wiccan and pagan cultures in the southern hemisphere, the cycle is amended, so celebrations can be worldwide, but with different seasonal observances. So, at this date in Australia, for example, it is the festival of Beltane.

nections in myth and legend about the Underworld, spirits, and ancestors.

In many cultures, it was thought that one's ancestors and loved ones who had passed on could visit during this time, often people would prepare their favourite meal or leave out treats for the spirits and souls. Candles were lit as a way to honour the departed, the guiding light in the window helping the spirits find their way back home. However, as the spirit world was inhabited by all kinds of beings, one may also disguise oneself with mask and costume in protection from more nefarious characters. One might prefer to keep safe and warm with feasting and games at home, repel dark spirits with protective charms and customs, or bravely seize the opportunity to perhaps face the fear of spirits and the dark by telling stories, dressing up as these beasts and making fun of what was feared.

Halloween is celebrated in many ways, under many names around Northern Europe, and now around the world. We'll find Allantide and *Kalan Gwav* in Cornwall, Hollantide in Wales and Isle of Man, and *Kala-Goanv* in Breton, All Hallows and Winternights...

All Hallows

The names Samhain and Halloween come from different roots but share a seasonal energy of moving into darkness. All Saints Day, also known as All Hallows' Day, was a day for the Church to remember those killed for their Christian beliefs at the end of the Roman Empire. It was originally celebrated in the spring, however, in the middle of the eighth century, it was moved from May 13th to November 1st. The night before All Hallows' Day then became known as "All Hallows' Eve," which was then shortened to "Hallowe'en." On these hallowed days (hallow meaning honoured as holy), church bells rang all night to ward off evil spirits, people lit candles and prayed for their dead. In many ways, I think Samhain harmonises quite nicely with these hallowed days by bringing in further ideas of the end of a cycle.

Winternights

In pre-Christian Scandinavia, the end of October was the time of Winternights, a three-day festival to start the dark winter season and honour both ancestral spirits and the spirits of the land. Winternights combines the celebration of the onset of winter with a harvest festival and honouring of the dead. The last sheaves of corn may be left in offering to Odin, and rituals are led by women to bless the household and all within. In some customs, the

Wild Hunt begin their ride now and continue to ride all through winter until spring. This warning of hellish fiends wandering in the night was a reminder to draw homewards, safely away from the cold and harsh weather. Work moved from fields and into the home in crafts and preparation for the long nights and Winternights brought light and joy to the season, with festivities and kinship: tales were told, great deeds and battles toasted.

Irish Samhain

In Ireland, when the harvest was brought in, a few stalks had to be left behind, this was the *púca's* share (*púca* being a ghost or nature spirit) and must be left to appease them. On Samhain a small offering might also be left out for the *púca*. In many parts of Ireland, a fruit cake called *barm brack* is served, inside which symbolic items are hidden: a ring for marriage, a coin for wealth...*barm brack* would also be handed out to those 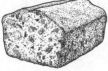 calling at your home at this time. Visitors on this night may well be on a journey visiting houses "mumming" or "guising" (as in, disguise) where people dress in costume with faces smudged from bonfire soot, either as protection or mimicry of the supernatural forces at large during Samhain.

Cornish Allantide

Like many traditions connected to Halloween, the coming of winter was associated with mortality and spirits in Cornwall. During the festivities, church bells may be tolled to aid the passage of the spirits.

This celebration in Cornwall included gifting apples as symbols of good luck. As well as enjoying eating these shiny apples, children might play games like Snap Apple or place the apple under their pillow at night for a foresight into the future; girls might hope for a vision of a prospective husband.

A specific kind of large, sweet red apple was most popular, called the Allan apple. And Halloween was often called Allantide, Allan Apple day or the Feast of St. Allan after the apple, but also associations with the local holy figure of St. Allan/Allen (it's not clear if the saint or the apple came first!).

Something of an obscure saint, little is known of St. Allen, except that, he may have been a sixth-century bishop from France. However, as M. A. Courtney reminds us in *Cornish Feasts and Folk-lore*, "there are more saints in Cornwall than there are in heaven." The likes of St. Allen, St. Austell, St. Piran and St. Levan seem to exist largely in Cornwall alone.

You can still find Allantide celebrations in rural villages in Cornwall and some of the larger towns that attract tourists, such as Penzance and St. Ives, enjoyed by tourists and locals alike; the festivities continue to bring people together, and offer a chance to share and retell stories and folklore.

Breton Celebrations

If we follow Celtic communities over to France, this time was known as *Kala-Goanv* to the Breton community. (In Cornwall some still know Samhain as *Kalan Gwav*, meaning "first day of winter." So you can see how various names and customs of Celtic practice have travelled through communities with slight variations.)

Leading up to November, stags fight and clash their antlers together, and Kala-Goanv marks the end of this time as the deer lose their antlers. (Stags and antlers can be seen in many European and Celtic artifacts, giving a strong hint as to the importance of these animals and stag-like deities through Europe.)

This was a time when ancestral spirits were thought to enter the world of the living, hungry for sustenance, so food is set aside for them in offering. Candles were lit in hollowed out beetroots and *cornigou* (little horn cakes) were baked by women to celebrate the season.

Pumpkins, Turnips and Jack-o'-Lanterns

One of the most familiar symbols of modern Halloween is the glowing orange face of a carved pumpkin. But where did this tradition come from?

There is an old Irish myth about a blacksmith, Stingy Jack. Jack was a blacksmith who tricked the Devil.[*] He offered his soul in exchange for a drink, but as the Devil turns himself into a sixpence to pay the bartender, Jack traps him in his pocket until he promises not to claim Jack's soul for ten years. The Devil agrees, but ten years later, Jack plays a similar trick and traps the Devil in an apple tree, releasing him for another promise not to claim Jack's soul.

But this means that when Jack dies, he is denied entrance into both heaven and hell: God not wanting unsavoury figures

---

[*] Folk tales about blacksmiths and devils are considered to be some of the oldest fairy tales in Europe.

in heaven, and the Devil having promised not to take his soul (and he's still upset by the tricks Jack had played on him).

So, the Devil sends Jack off into the dark night with only a lump of burning coal from the fires of hell to light his way. Depending on the telling, Jack hollows out a turnip or cabbage to carry the ember and give him light and has been roaming the earth ever since. This ghostly figure was called "Jack of the Lantern," which in time was shortened to "Jack-o'-lantern," and this story was remembered each year by carving faces on vegetables and placing a burning piece of coal inside.

When Irish immigrants arrived in America in the 1840s, they took their Samhain/Halloween traditions with them, including the tradition of carving-out turnips. They quickly discovered however, that Jack-o'-lanterns were much easier to carve out of the pumpkin, which was a fruit native to their newly-adopted American home. So, in time, pumpkins replaced turnips, and candles replaced the burning coals. And because of the legend of Jack, for hundreds of years, people have put carved vegetables with candles in their window to scare away any malevolent wandering souls or evil spirits.

To the modern Kitchen Witch, the pumpkin may symbolise protection; abundance as harvest foodstuff; hope as a light in the dark; and transformation from foodstuff to magical lantern (and then back into food again if you chop up the lantern and put it into a soup!).

Apples and Nuts

Really, thought Poirot, one didn't seem able to get away from apples. Nothing could be more agreeable than a juicy English apple – and yet here were apples mixed up with broomsticks, and witches, and old-fashioned folklore..."
Agatha Christie, *Hallowe'en Party* (1969)

Bobbing for apples (also known as apple bobbing, dunking for apples, ducking, duck-apple or dooking) – a game in which apples float in a tub of water and are retrieved using only one's mouth – was once something young people played at Halloween parties to seek the destiny of their love life: each apple might be assigned to a potential suitor, and the bobber might try to bite into the apple named for their favourite. Another version was that the first to bite an apple would be the first to marry. After the apples were retrieved from the water, they might be peeled and long segments of skin could reveal the first initial of a future spouse. Or the bobbed apple could be placed underneath one's pillow to reveal a future soulmate in dream. Apple bobbing is still popular today amongst children at Halloween parties, though without the divination element.

You may have heard the term "Snap Apple Night" as a synonym for Halloween. In the game of Snap Apple, an apple was speared on one end of a stick while lit candles were fixed around it; the stick was spun around, and the participants' goal was to take a bite of the apple, avoiding a face full of hot wax! Another fire-themed game was Snapdragon, where raisins are soaked in brandy and set aflame, the game is to pull the raisins from the flames without burning yourself!

Another food-based name for Halloween is "Nut-crack Night," inspired by other fortune-telling customs popular at Samhain and Yuletide in Northern England and Scotland. As the chill of autumn drew in, people might sit around their fires eating hazelnuts or chestnuts or throwing them into the fire. One might give each nut a value (like yes or no, 'loves me' or 'loves me not'), or the name of a possible sweetheart and watch to see which burned the brightest, or cracked first as an indicator of an answer. Or observing the movement of the nuts as drawing closer or moving apart from one another.

Two hazelnuts I threw into the flame,
And to each nut I gave a sweetheart's name:
This with the loudest bounce me sore amazed,
That is a flame of brightest colour blazed;
As blazed the nut, so may thy passion grow,
For 'twas thy nut that did so brightly glow!

John Gay, "The Spell" (early 1700s)

Based somewhere in these games and jollities were hidden the real practices of witches and cunning folk, of using foods such as apples and nuts in divination. These are skills that ancient and modern witches, mediums and oracles use with varying amounts of success.

Honouring the Dead

Dumb Suppers and Sin Eaters

There is something invaluable and healing about remembering those we have lost and deliberately inviting their presence into our lives and family occasions. It can help both commemorate and grieve a loss, but also to cross between memory and the present moment.

Many cultures mark this time of year by honouring their dead with offerings of food and flowers. Those who believed that the dead visit the living on this night may leave food out for them at home or on family graves as offerings. The concept of leaving food for spirit ancestors and the dead is ancient.

The ritual of "the dumb supper" – found through parts of Europe and North America –memorialises and honours the dead. Participants set the table with a place for the dead and meals often contain the favourite foods of the departed. There are variants where the dumb supper takes place at midnight, but for others, it is a meal taken at dusk, a liminal time. The dumb supper was intended to encourage the appearance of a spirit, not unlike a seance. Fires and candles may be lit, and doors left open to help guide them inside.

In America, a variation is that the meal is eaten backwards, with dessert first and each place setting opposite of what it normally is. This could be connected to enduring ideas of practices of the occult and magical being about inversion in some way, like images of witches riding brooms and animals backwards.

Dumb Cakes and Soul Cakes

There are many links between cakes and divination. In England and Scotland, many young women would have baked special "dumb cakes," either as part of a dumb supper or alone, to be eaten in silence in order to invite a future husband to appear in her dreams.

Cakes have been used by people all over the world to honour their dead. Earlier in the book we learned about the Italian *fave dei morti*, "beans of the dead" biscuits, eaten at this time of year. The practice of baking a soul cake or soulmass cake to commemorate and celebrate the dead for Halloween, All Saints' Day and All Souls' Day in England dates back at least to the medieval period (which is usually when the first records appear, so it is understood that traditions date long before that too). These small, round, spiced cakes were given out to children and the poor who often went door to door to seek food and favour in return for prayers and songs, in a practice called "souling." In this (along with the customs of mumming and guising) we can see the roots of our modern custom of trick or treating.

The Kitchen Witch's Hedgerow and Garden

To discover something, pick it, take it home and make something beautiful out of it, jam to glisten on shelves through winter, is the most elementary form of magic. You are providing for yourself, bottling summer to see you through the darkest times. You are trapping sunlight in with the sugar, to unscrew when the days are hung rain and biting wind.

Alice Tarbuck, *A Spell in the Wild* (2020)

Notes on the *Witch's* Hedgerow

Part of the joy of foraging or observing your local hedgerows is tuning into the rhythm and seasons of your particular area. If you live in the luscious far south of the British Isles or Europe you may enjoy fruits sooner in the year, and if you are of the beautiful north of this region you may need to wait a little longer for your hedgerow bounty, and appreciate it all the more. All manner of variables will have an effect. But if you take regular visits into nature, you will find you can begin to connect and predict the ripening of certain fruits and berries. Some may call you a witch for that, this is our glorious ability to find connection to nature, use mindful attention, and our own intuition.

This is the season of red berries, brown nuts and changing leaves of golden hues. Ruby rosehips, rowan and hawthorn berries may be found dotted in the hedges or woodland through into midwinter.

Remember the blossoms of Ostara and Beltane? We are at the wheels opposite point now at Samhain, and those apple blossoms are now ripe fruits, which will be a mainstay of the coming months. Hazelnuts and walnuts are decadent treats for the forager.

Hazelnuts, when fully ripe, drop from their husks, although they're also edible when they're fresh and green, we have always called these cobb nuts in my family.

It is no coincidence that the things we associate with traditional Halloween celebrations – pumpkins, turnips, apples, and nuts – were all nature's bounty, recently harvested from gardens and farms. Even in these days of buckets of factory-made sweets being handed out to children trick or treating, we still retain these threads (and treats) of Halloween's past.

Kitchen Witch Celebrations for Samhain

With these seasonal festivals comes a sense of mystery, magic, and stories that many more than just witches and pagans can enjoy. Everyone can enjoy the light, warmth and scents of a bonfire and the joyful light of fireworks, of candles lit on windowsills and in carved pumpkins, of caramelised apples and spiced hot libations. And note, as we look through these practices, yes, there are connections with the dead, but also how often the traditions are about love: some traditions for seeking out love, and some celebrating lost love and departed loved ones.

So bake the soul cakes, and harvest the apples, light the candles and celebrate love! Dine with joy and in memory. And invite the spirits in if you wish. For winter is nearing, and soon enough the bright lights of Yule will be on their way...

Notes on Celebration

Like the hedgerow, the best advice is to go outside in your local region and see what's happening. If you are able, seek out the local customs in your area. The ones that date back so far no one can quite remember why they are done perhaps (though many a local will have some stories to tell). These traditions are kept alive with joy and merriment: flaming tar barrels and clavies, cheese rolling, Jack-in-the-green and chimney sweeps parades, the Mari Lwyd horses of Wales and hobby horses prancing through Cornwall as well as many blessings of ploughs, fleets, sheaves and fishing nets.

Celebrating Today

☾ Gather in the last of the harvest: apples, squashes, pumpkins, nuts and by the power of your kitchen magic they become cakes, jams, soups, stews and warming delights.

☾ Apples carefully stored, can last in a cool dark place till Imbolc.

☾ Bake your own soul cakes, perhaps make them part of a dumb supper.

☾ Try your hand at divination with nuts or apples.

☾ Carve a pumpkin or turnip. Light up your Jack-o'-Lantern in October and turn it into a warming soup for November!

☾ Invite friends around for a Samhain party, dress up, play games and share stories.

WINTER SOLSTICE AND YULE

The process of coming into the dark that started at the Autumn Equinox and Samhain, reaches its peak at Winter Solstice, the shortest day of the year, and consequently, longest night, also known as Yule to many pagans and witches.

We know from Palaeolithic monuments like Stonehenge that our ancient ancestors honoured the Winter Solstice in some way with ritual, fires and food. The word "Yule" arrived in Britain with the Germanic invasion around the eleventh century, with varying ideas about its exact definition, but drawn from common roots: *Jul* in Sweden, Denmark, and Norway, *Jól* in Iceland and the Faroe Islands, *Joelfeest* in the Netherlands. Perhaps with connections to the Old Norse word *hjól* meaning "wheel" and signifying winter as an extreme point of the year's cycle.

The Yule festivals were understandably very important to these northernmost European cultures, recipients of some of the darkest and harshest winters. For the Anglo-Saxons, the word Christmas (*Cristes maesse*, Christ's Mass) appeared in use around 1038. Before that it was simply the time of "midwinter" and the longest night, Winter Solstice, was called *Modranacht*, Mother Night, a chance perhaps to connect to female ancestors and acknowledge the primaeval darkness that will bear the new year.

In the harsh winter weather there are no crops to gather, no ground to till, preserving and bottling has been done and animals are in their winter shelters and so most work carried on indoors: knitting, sewing, woodworking, weaving, mending, candle making... Though not idle, there may have been a little more opportunity of rest whilst staying warm inside. Midwinter offered a transformation from everyday toil to turn attention toward festivities. For the wealthy, this would be a season of abundance, parties and light; to the poor, it may be a time for a little more food, charity, merriment and time off from work to spend with the family.

Twelve Merry Days

One Yule tradition, still familiar to us today, though now in chocolate cake form, is the Yule log. Traditionally logs would be burnt in recognition and appeal to the return of the sun. Feasting and merriment would continue as long as the log burned. In a popular quote from the Norse text, *Heimskringla,* in the Saga of Hákon, the Good King of Norway said of Yule that toasts were to be drunk to the gods, for good harvests, for peace and to the memory of departed kinsfolk. People were counselled to "keep the holiday while the ale lasted."

Christmas and Christ's birthday was formally laid out by the Church in Rome as December 25th somewhere in the mid-fourth century. "Pagan" Romans already celebrated around the Winter Solstice, with Saturnalia celebrations lasting about a week celebrating the god Saturn, and deities of the sun. And they honoured the new year with the help of God Janus, who gifted his name to the month of January. With his two faces, he can look back to the old year, and onwards to the new year. As we are aware, Christmas would slowly take over and we would lose Saturnalia and similar festivals to history.

The twelve days, as Christians outlined it, take us neatly from Christmas day through New Year's Day to the Twelfth Night (January 5th). A twelve-day break from work and for celebrations were enshrined in law by King Alfred the Great in 877 CE. Throughout medieval and Tudor England (1066–1603), the twelve days off at Christmas and Yule were – just as the earth stood still – a chance to be idle. The lower classes that worked the land had less to do, and the upper classes enjoyed a chance to show off and feast.

The central part of Christmas was hospitality to family, friends and charity, often blending pagan and Christian traditions. Entertainment occurred in pubs, streets, in the big houses, and mummers (silent masked performers) might parade from house to house, performing in return for food. For the upper classes, these twelve days were a celebration of gifts, feasting, sweets and misrule, starting on Christmas day and culminating in the Twelfth Night climax of a grand banquet, often including spiced cakes, mince pies, and gingerbread.

During the 1640s and 1650s, Oliver Cromwell and the Puritans started heavily controlling Christmas church services, celebratory feasting and various elements of Christmas fun in England. Puritans were strongly against Christmas, deeming it too pagan and full of gluttony and drunkenness. Christmas was not banned completely, but all the best bits were, and with the risk that Christmas geese and mince pies could be confiscated by law, many festivities had to be a bit more clandestine! King Charles II restored Christmas when he ascended the throne in 1660, but not all the traditions of the twelve days came back when it was reinstated. Festivities can and do change through generations, but the main themes of this celebration are timeless – bringing light and warmth, feasting, merriment and thinking of others.

Winter festivities help us journey through these darkest days of the year. Revelling in fine foods and the company in which you eat them. Winter feasting is very special, as hot and plentiful food is all the more appreciated when it is scarce (as opposed to a midsummer feast when it may be in abundance!). In many cultures midwinter/Yule/Christmas still reign supreme as the days of feasting! Even now, when most of us can feast every day if we so wish, still we look forward to festive indulgences.

Festive Drinks

Mulled Wine
Mulled drinks – warmed with both spices and heat – are associated with Christmas, from German *Glühwein* (meaning glow wine) served at Christmas markets today, to mulled cider and apple juice in England. The Swedish version of mulled wine, *glogg*, is served with blanched almonds and raisins. Spices were added to preserve but also mask cheap alcohol or wine past its best. Recipes vary, but mulling spice mixtures tend to include orange peel, cloves, cinnamon and sometimes cardamom and star anise...as well as a good measure of sugar and a splash of a spirit. In Scotland you may enjoy Yule Ale, made

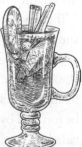

specially for Yule, not mulled per say, but ginger and treacle were added to the hops for a sweet, warming mix.

The practice of heating and spicing wines dates back at least to ancient Rome and Greece where herbs added flavour and healing properties.

Wassailing

Here we come a-wassailing
Among the leaves so green,
Here we come a-wand'ring
So fair to be seen.
Love and joy come to you,
And to you your wassail, too,
And God bless you, and send you
A Happy New Year.

"Wassail Song"

Wassail: Is it a warm libation? A ritual? A hearty salutation? A song? Why, it's all of these things! And it's rooted in traditions branching out for over a millennium, bringing merriment and mischief to the dark days of midwinter. The word "wassail" is drawn from the Anglo-Saxon phrase *"waes hael,"* which means "be well" or "be in good health." The word as we know it today appears in the poem "Beowulf" (1000 CE-ish) as a salute to warriors. Then, in 1135, Geoffrey of Monmouth told the story of Saxon princess, Rowena. She presents the British king, Vortigern with a bowl of spiced wine, saluting him with a *"Wass-heil!"* to which he answered, *"Drinc heile!"* and quite taken with her charms, he later marries her.

There is no definitive recipe for wassail, as it varies from county to county and was often dependant on local ingredients, but you'll usually find plentiful apples involved. The wassail drink has been made of warm beer, ale or cider, cloves, ginger, nutmeg and sugar, sometimes with bread, cake or sliced apples floating in it and pulped roasted apples known as "Lamb's Wool." It may also be fortified by wine, brandy, whisky, rum, or in fact, any alcoholic liquid provided by revellers (like many a mystery punch at parties you may have been to!). Varied as the ingredients may have been, the mixture would have been sweet, hot and boozy, with one or two warming and healing herbs or spices. Wassail, the drink, is offered to visitors and becomes a social activity when taken around the village in a bowl decorated with evergreen leaves (usually holly and ivy) and garlands of red ribbons. Along with the drink would be a range of festive customs that might also include singing, jokes and guessing games.

Wassail, wassail, all over the town;
Our toast it is white, our ale it is brown,
Our bowl it is made of the mapling tree;
With the wassailing bowl we will drink to thee.

Another Wassail song, this one was found in *A Right Merrie Christmas: The Story of Christ-tide* by John Ashton (1894)

The wassailing ritual of blessing trees and singing through the town is done all through Yuletide, depending on the area and traditions. Taking the wassail out to the local orchards in ritual was intended to ensure an abundant apple harvest as well as wishing good health to others in the community. It is also meant to scare away any evil spirits that might be lurking in the branches, and in some regions, men fire guns, and people bang on pots and pans for the same effect. The toast or cake floating in the mixture is sometimes hung up in the trees as well as a sort of offering, literally "raising a toast," into the boughs of the trees to feed and thank the trees for giving apples. Wassailers might make rounds of their village and wassail fields, livestock and even visit beehives to declare "Waes Hael!" to the bees, to assure abundance for the coming year. This ritual of wassail is still prevalent in my home counties of Somerset and Wiltshire, places famous for their apple orchards, including the mythical orchards of Avalon.[*]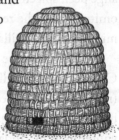

There are many studies connected to wassailing from the respectable likes of the Royal Horticultural Society which show that kind words and even songs directed at plants can affect their growth. So, as funny as practices like this may seem to us today, there is never any harm in wishing the trees well!

---

[*]   There are certainly many apple orchards in the area, and those remaining are owned and protected by the National Trust, who suggest Glastonbury was named Avalon in the Iron Age because of the treasured apple orchards (Avalon means 'the isle of apples').

Puddings and Pies

The Christmas pudding (also known as figgy pudding and plum pudding) is a rich and hearty boiled pudding still served today in the UK and Ireland on Christmas Day after a Christmas dinner of roast turkey or goose. In the past it would only have been enjoyed by wealthier families who had access to luxuries such as dried fruits and oranges from the Mediterranean and exotic spices, sugar and rum.

Inside a Christmas pudding one may find small coins that are supposed to bring wealth and good luck to whoever finds them, or a bean, which would dictate who would become the Lord of Misrule for the day. This was a treasured part of the Tudor Twelve Days of Christmas, the act of turning things on their heads, making fools into kings for a day, and servants into masters.

English Lord of Misrule traditions may be drawn from (or loosely connected to) similar Roman midwinter traditions of Saturnalia: festivities that included normal orders of things reversed, and accepted etiquettes abandoned. To oversee events, a king or a master of ceremonies would issue games and outlandish instructions.

Mince pies, another traditional English treat eaten only at Christmas, have been through quite a few forms. Pies made with spices and meat appear in English texts dating back to 1390, and they have featured everything from finely minced meat and chopped fruit such as raisins, prunes, dates, and orange peel, spiced with cloves, mace, and cinnamon. Over time, the meat was omitted from the recipe and just suet (meat fat) used, resulting in the fruity mix that is so familiar today, and still known as mincemeat.

Along with recipe changes, name changes have known mince pies also as Christmas pies (indicating their popularity at this time of year), shred pies (referring to the shredded suet and meat) and wayfarer's pies (as a treat served to travelling visitors.) A warm mince pie was a luxury in the dark, stormy winter months. Today they are still served at festive parties, and of course, left on the fireplace by children for Father Christmas when he calls with presents on Christmas Eve.

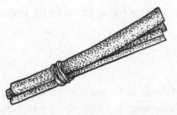

Stargazy Pie – Cornish Magic

Almost anything under the sun may be put into a pie, and no one be the wiser, for the crust puts on a brave face and hides the poverty (should there be poverty) underneath. No end of stories have been told of pies... Old Nick comes in and watches a woman make an "all-sorts" pie, in which nothing seemed out of place, and so afraid was he that his own dear self would be included that he skipped out of the county. The pie, like the pasty, is a mystery until it is opened, unless the crust is decorated with the foot of a duck or some other indication of contents. The heads of pilchards peeping through the crust suggested the name of "star-gazey pie."

J. Henry Harris, *Cornish Saints and Sinners* **(1906)**

I now had the delightful opportunity of once more breathing my native air, viewing beautiful Mount Edgcumbe, revelling in clotted cream and potted pilchards, tickling my palate...with John-dories, conger eels, star-gazey and squab pies.

A Sailor of King George: The Journals of Captain Frederick Hoffman **(1793–1814)**

In terms of niche tales from small places, stargazy pie is special as a distinctly Cornish Christmas food: it features the heads and tails of pilchards which poke out of a pastry lid, so they can gaze skyward, with their bodies tucked under the pastry.

In Cornwall's tiny port town of Mousehole, many years ago (depending on the tale, it can date back to the sixteenth century) winter storms were thrashing the village. None of the fishing boats were able to leave the harbour on such rough seas, and the village was cut off. The people were starving, so a local man called Tom Bowcock bravely sailed out into the stormy seas and fished through the night, navigating by the few scarce stars that could be seen through the storm clouds, catching enough fish to feed the entire village. The whole catch went into pies, which had the fish heads poking out, maybe to prove that there were fish inside, or maybe so they could gaze at the stars that helped guide Tom's way home on that stormy night. Every year since then, in December, stargazy pie is cooked and eaten at The Ship Inn at Mousehole Harbour.

Gingerbread and Witches' Houses

Gingerbread houses are a traditional Christmas treat from Germany. Gingerbread itself is much older. It has connections to both ancient Greece and Egypt, and was introduced into Europe in the eleventh century as trading along the spice routes from the Middle East developed. It was popular for gingerbread dough to be pressed into moulds of kings, queens or religious symbols. While the first edible "gingerbread men" are often attributed to Queen Elizabeth I in the 1500s, this is likely just the first documented incident as she presented important visitors with biscuits baked in their own image.

Lebkuchen – a spiced cake containing ginger – is a centuries-old German spiced treat traditionally baked during the winter months. And to make elaborate brightly decorated houses, became closely tied with Christmas/Yule traditions. Popularity soared, however, when the Brothers Grimm wrote the story of "Hansel and Gretel," in which brother and sister stumble upon the house of a witch, made of sweet treats in a deep dark forest. This is likely where that alternative name for gingerbread houses in Germany came from: *"Hexenhaus"* (Witch's House).

In the first edition of "Hansel and Gretel" the witch's house was described as "a little house that was made entirely of bread and covered with cake, and the windows were made of light-coloured sugar."[19]

The actual "gingerbread house" would arrive in later versions of the story – along with embellishments in the retelling like decorations of icing sugar, cookies, chocolate, candy, and sweets (which may reflect real gingerbread houses seen at Yuletide). In most modern re-tellings of the story, the gingerbread house is a now crucial feature, like Perrault's Cinderella with her pumpkin coach and glass slipper – we may find it hard to imagine some classic tales without these key elements.

Building gingerbread houses became a popular pastime in Germany, and as *Lebkuchen*/gingerbread was already associated with Christmas, gingerbread houses became a very popular and recognisable symbol of the festive season throughout Germany, the rest of Northern Europe and beyond. And the ritual of creating and decorating the house is a sweet ritual in itself, often done as a family.

Light and Dark

The Hunt that falls between Christmas and Twelfth Day, when the su-
pernatural has sway, and wild beasts like the wolf are not mentioned by
their names, brings fertility to the land... At the same time Holda, like
Wuotan,[*] *can also ride on the winds, clothed in terror, and she, like the god,*
belongs to the 'wutende heer.[†] *From this arose the fancy, that witches ride in*
Holda's company...

Jacob Grimm, *Deutsche Mythologie* (1835)

In this, the darkest and stormiest time of the year in Northern European
countries, the sun barely rises, if at all, and the dead are said to return to earth,
seeking to share feasts with the living. But other magical creatures run freely
at this time too in The Wild Hunt – a cacophony of souls riding through the
sky; ghostly steeds, hounds, witches, demons, and deities dance over howling winds and raging storms. *The Anglo-Saxon Chronicles*[‡] described spectral
winter huntsmen as terrifying beings riding on black horses and goats, followed by terrible "wide-eyed" hounds. One may make an offering of food,
but others say if food is left out the Wild Hunt will whip through the house
and devour everything in it.

The Germanic version of "The Wild Hunt of Odin and Holda" lasted
twelve nights and was popularized by Jacob Grimm in his own collections of
stories and folklore.

Goddess Holda and Frau Holle

You may stay with me if you help me about the house. You must make my bed
and give it a good shake so the feathers fly. Then it will snow on earth, for I
am Frau Holle.

The Original Folk and Fairy Tales of the Brothers Grimm (1812)

The goddess Holda[§] goes by many names and identities: Mistress of Yule,

---

[*]   *Wodin/Odin*

[†]   *"Wutende heer"* means angry army or wild hunt.

[‡]   A collection of manuscripts written as diaries/annals by monks in England between the
ninth and twelfth centuries.

[§]   Jacob Grimm connected a lot of goddesses and women together in his work with a
dizzying array of different spellings and suggested that Holle, Holda, Perchta and Berchta
are all names for the same figure.

Stormbringer, Mother of Lost Souls, Weaver, Winter's White Crone, Bright One, Queen of the Witches, She who leads the wild band of lost souls and most commonly today, Frau Holle. She is visualised in many forms, pre-Christian deity, earth goddess, witch figure and fairy tale character.

As was the fate of many goddesses connected to female domestic crafts, Holda's link to spinning and weaving, and day-to-day tasks such as shaking out bedding, soon meant that she became associated with witchcraft. In some imagery she rides with witches on distaffs (a stick used in spinning). When she's not in flight, the *Hoher Meißner* (High Meissner) mountain in Germany is considered by many to be her home, amongst the old beech trees, wych elms and oaks. The folklore of Frau Holle has been brought to life on that mountain, at the edge of Frau Holle Pond stands a wooden statue of her, created in 2004. She holds in her hand a feather pillow ready to shake when she's ready to change the weather.

Just like Frau Holle, Holda, as the goddess of winter, brings the first snowflakes of the year, shaking out her goose-feather blankets until the feathers fall as snowflakes to the mortal world. She was also associated with other weather phenomena: when it rained, Holda was doing her washing; lightning was her scorching flax; the fog was the smoke from her chimney. Her association with winter ties into her role as goddess of the domestic arts and patroness of housewives, women and children. Echoing past goddesses who taught humans (namely women) household skills, it was the goddess Holda who first taught mortals the art of growing flax, spinning, and of weaving it, and it is a craft under her protection. Braided loaves called *Hollenzopf*, "Holles/Holdas braid" are sweet breads often baked at Yule in Germanic countries in homage to Holda's connections to braids of hair or thread, and loaves may well have been left out for her as she sweeps through households at Yule to make sure all is in order.

As winter is traditionally a time to work on all the homecrafts overseen by the goddess – weaving, cleaning, brewing, baking, cooking – perhaps every Kitchen Witch who has found magic in the arts of the home has entered into Holda's realm.

The Bright Ones – Perchta/Berchta

Perchta is a goddess from the German and Austrian regions of the Alps whose name may originate from the Old High German word *peraht* ("brilliant" or "bright") in some places she is Perchta, others call her Berchta. She, like

Holda (and she is often thought to be a regional variation of this goddess), is known to examine the spinning rooms and homestead to make sure they are in good order, and that no work is done over sacred Yuletide. But (and things take a dark turn here) if these are a real mess or anyone in the household has not eaten *Zemmede*[*] that day, she'll slit open your belly and fill it with straw and stones!

Although possibly the same figure, in some lore it seems that Perchta is the more devilish incarnation and Berchta is a kindlier, crone figure so ancient a saying in some parts of France and Europe referred to an event from long past as "from the time when Berchta used to spin." The contrasting faces of these folkloric figures may have been a representation of dual personalities, or perhaps Christianity slowly turning these figures from goddesses and sorceresses to demons and fearsome witches.

One custom that still exists today in the mountains of Austria is the *"Perchtenlauf"* – Perchta's entourage. In an adoption of Wild Hunt themes, a masked parade of people dressed as beasts with large horns (a symbol that also connects to the image of the *Krampus* – a devilish looking festive demon that punishes the naughty, possibly the masculine form of Perchta) served to frighten away the cold and the evil spirits of winter. Also known as *Rauhnacht* – night of smoke – it is common for children to go from house to house, asking for a cakes and sweets as part of the festivities.

Saffron Buns, Saints and Witches
On St. Lucia's Day, December 13th, in Sweden (and other areas of Scandinavia), it is customary for the eldest daughter of a household to dress as St. Lucia in a white robe and a crown of nine candles (traditionally the crown is made with whortleberry or lingonberry twigs). She wakes up the family with fresh coffee and golden saffron buns – *lussebullar* – in her honour. These saffron buns are baked into many different shapes, but the one you may see most often is a curling S shape that mimics the circled shape of a cat's tail called *lussekatter* "Lucia's Cats."

St. Lucia (or St. Lucy) is, to Christians, a martyr, best known for her crown of candles and offering up food. In some tales, she brings food down into

---

[*]   According to Grimm, Perchta demands that certain meals be consumed and offered to her on her feast day. *Zemmede* is a mix of flour, milk, and water and baked in a pan. (Sounds like we're back to pancakes again!)

caves and catacombs where Christians are hiding, led by candles which she places in a crown around her head so that her hands are free to carry food. In others, she stands at the helm of a brilliant white boat on the longest night of the year and distributes food to starving villagers.

Honoured as a light-bringer, her feast represents light overcoming darkness and her name Lucia/Lucy comes from the Latin *lux*, meaning light. There are hints that Lucia comes from pagan origins. Some link her to sun goddesses, and others with Holda and Perchta. Jacob Grimm suggested that Berchta, was potentially linked to St Lucia of Sweden. There are some big differences certainly, but the presence of light-bringing on dark winter nights does connect them.

Some connect Lucia with stories of a witch called Lussi, who leads the procession of *Lussiferda* (a word my search engine and spell check desperately wanted to 'correct' to Lucifer). A lot like the Wild Hunt, this entourage of demons and witches flies over the night sky on December 13th. Lussi's horde destroyed chimneys if certain tasks weren't done: spinning of thread or yarn and cleaning had to be finished, preserving meats, and other such tasks you'd need to help you survive through winter (this is very similar to the story of goddess Holda and her own Wild Hunt).

Winter Solstice in Norway, is often known as *Lussia Langnatte* (or Lussi's Long Night). In Sweden its *Lussinatta* (Lussi's Night) and many folk traditions connect to both the saintly image of Lucia and the more demonic Lussi. (Prior to the 1700s, when calendar reforms shifted things around a bit, December 13th was the Winter Solstice, hence the association with the coming of the light.) To mark the event, one might practice *Lussevaka* and stay awake through the night to guard oneself and the household against evil and celebrate the passing of a long winter's night by cooking and making the *lussekatter* rolls to eat come morning.

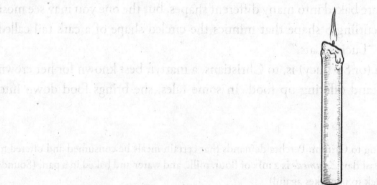

Tomte

Tomte (from Swedish, *tonttu* in Finnish, *nisse* in Danish) are house spirits – *tomte* translates as "homestead man" – responsible for the protection and welfare of a farmstead and its buildings.

The *tomte* tend to be associated with Yuletide, perhaps because he is often depicted as a very short and very strong, elderly bearded man with a red cap... But also, because he often helps out preparing the home for Christmas. He seems to watch over the home in a way the Kitchen Witch poppet would admire! Believed by some to be the soul of the farm's first owner, who becomes a spirit figure to watch over it, *tomtes* are valuable guardians – but payment is always required for their loyalty. One must respect the *tomte*, treat your farm and animals well, and at Yuletide, offer food as thanks for their protection throughout the year. On Christmas Eve, Swedish children leave out a bowl of Yule rice pudding flavoured with cinnamon and sugar, butter or cream at the front door for the *tomte*. If the bowl is found empty the next morning, the year ahead will be prosperous.

A sure way to incur the anger of a *tomte* is rudeness and untidiness, and if you were to spill anything on the kitchen floor, it is polite to shout a warning to the *tomte* lest he fall into the spillage.

The Kitchen Witch's Hedgerow and Garden

At first glance, there may seem little to be found in the hedgerow at this time of year except evergreen plants, the red berries of holly and white of mistletoe. Trees have shed their leaves and frost sparkles on dawn grasses. Morning hazes hang heavy over the valleys, taking longer to dissipate on cold mornings.

But food can still be found if you know where to look. Winter flavours are rich, dark and earthy: chestnuts, mushrooms, and winter squashes. Amongst the frosted hedgerows, the glow of crimson rosehips might still be seen in December, and sloes are thought to be at their best when picked just after the first frost. We can seek fungi, including oyster mushrooms and winter chanterelles, in woodlands. You may also find in the British Isles the festive sounding snowy waxcaps and scarlet elf cups. Whilst looking on the woodland floor, keep a keen eye for sweet chestnuts, a treat when roasted to bring out their sweet nutty taste. Chestnuts are a perennially popular Christmas food, especially at Christmas markets and outdoor festive events where you can smell the roasted nuts warming on little carts. Look out for their spiny casings on the ground amongst the leaves of the winter woodland floor, you can roast them at home and eat warm. If you have any left, they are a treat as part of Christmas stuffing.

Kitchen Witch Celebrations for Yule

In the past, the winter dark would have held some trepidation and anxiety: a multitude of unknowns could leave people starving and freezing. Although survival is less of a question now for most of us, there are still challenges of getting up in the dark, battling inclement weather, and the low light levels that can cause a lack of vitamin D and seasonal depression.

Much of folklore sees winter and the dark nights with a sense of apprehension: to be approached mindfully. And with this energy of mindfulness, we have an invitation to explore.

What does the dark of winter bring up for you? Where can you shine light in the darkness? What could you let fall away like the dry winter leaves from a tree? What are you trying to keep up that is more draining than joyful? How might you rest and create cosiness in celebration of the long dark nights? This is a wonderful time to light candles and use warming incense or essential oils (I'm looking at you cinnamon and clove!) to wrap up warm on windy, rainy nights with music and a book, games with friends or sitting in circle and telling stories. We can in our own way, enjoy and embrace a little hibernation in winter.

Celebrating Today

(So many ideas for baking! You might be inspired to try mince pies, saffron buns, stargazy pie, Christmas cake or pudding, a gingerbread house or pancakes for Perchta.

(Make a chocolate Yule log...or burn a real one if you have a fireplace or woodburning stove.

(Wassail what is dear to you: people, trees, bees...whatever you wish!

(Gather evergreen winter plants – holly, ivy, eucalyptus, spruce – to make a wreath or garland for your door, or to decorate your home.

(Brew up some mulled wine or juice and celebrate the season with friends.

(Discard guilt about seeking soothing, nourishing foods: warm stews, baked breads, butter, honey, cream, rice puddings, hot buns, and hot coffee. They fuel and warm you in more ways than one, enjoy this food for heart and soul.

NEW YEAR AND TWELFTH NIGHT

New Year's Eve (December 31st), New Year's Day (January 1st) and Twelfth Night, January 6th (also known as Epiphany, marking the arrival of the Three Kings to visit the baby Jesus) would have once been, and to many still are, the most important part of the festivities of the winter festivals.

Hogmanay

With the arrival of the Protestant Reformation to Scotland in 1560 and their extreme dislike of fripperies and festivities and Yule vacations, *"Christ's mass"* was abolished. Christmas only became a bank holiday in Scotland in 1958, so for many, Hogmanay on December 31st is the bigger festival, with deep roots in Scottish folklore. Hogmanay, New Year's night, was often known as *Oidhche Choinnle* – Candle Night. It saw candles lit and fires kept burning all night inside and outside of the home. Great care was taken to keep these fires alive, for if they went out, no one would give out coals for a new fire. It was considered to be unlucky to give away anything connected to fuel or abundance, and might even invite harmful sorcery. So, in keeping the fire alive and treasures close, any evil was kept away from the house for the following year.

Immediately after midnight one may well sing Robert Burns' "Auld Lang Syne" popular through Scotland and British Isles. Auld Lang Syne, means *times long past* or *days gone by*. So the song is about coming together, remembering friends and raising a glass for the sake of old times, and is often sung in circle holding hands.

Should auld acquaintance be forgot and never brought to mind?
Should auld acquaintance be forgot and auld lang syne
For auld lang syne, my dear, for auld lang syne,
We'll take a cup o' kindness yet, for auld lang syne.

After the Hogmanay celebrations of feasting, songs and fires, and midnight has chimed, attentions turn to the first person to enter the house. Known as the "first-foot", it was most important for the luck of the household in the coming year that they should not make their entry empty-handed. They should cross the threshold with symbolic gifts such as salt, coal, shortbread, and whisky so that the house should not want for these provisions through the coming year. First footers may be offered a "Het Pint" a hot pint made from spiced ale, nutmeg, sugar, eggs, and other spirits. It might be offered to visitors or carried in copper kettles by first-footers on their rounds through the neighbourhood and offered up to those they meet.

New Year's Day, was considered a great saining day. The woman of the house would go from room to room with a smouldering juniper branch, filling the house with purifying smoke to bless and protect the home and land, after which the windows would be thrown open and reviving drams of whisky would be passed around.

Women's Christmas

Still celebrated in Ireland on January 6th, and often known as Little Christmas, *Nollaig na mBan* (Women's Christmas) was the day that women, who have been in charge of all the Christmas cooking and festivities in the home, get a well-deserved break. Women do not cook dinner on this day, instead the men are left in charge of house and children and the women head out to the bars or friends' homes to drink, chat and let their hair down. Usually a raucous occasion, it is a brave man who shows his face in the pub that night![20]

Epiphany – La Befana – The Good Witch
In Italian folklore, the witch of Christmas would definitely be described as a good witch. La Befana is the witch who brings good children treats on the

morning of the Epiphany, January 6th.

La Befana has, by some, been woven into the Christmas tale of Christ's birth. It is said that after refusing to join the Wise Men on their journey to see the baby Jesus, she regrets her decision and sets out alone to bring gifts to the holy child, but never finds him. Instead, she leaves gifts for other children.

Italian children might write wishes on slips of paper to send up the chimney to La Befana and leave out their shoes or put up stockings on Epiphany eve. She flies around the world on a broomstick and comes down chimneys to deliver tangerines, candies, chocolates and presents to children who have been good during the year. For those who have been bad, La Befana will leave lumps of coal, sticks or dark candy – some shops in Italy sell black rock candy that actually look like pieces of coal for this occasion! Being a good housekeeper, she may well use her broom to sweep the floor before she leaves, sweeping away the problems of the past year. A family may leave a glass of wine and a plate of food to help fuel her travels. And all kinds of Befana cakes and cookies are made across Italy; in some regions, La Befana's arrival is celebrated with a panettone fruit bread; in others, a star-shaped bread called focaccia della Befana is made.

Another Story of an Italian Good Witch and of Coal

A *strega** named Arima once lived in Milan. In the small area of the city around Via Laghetto, behind the great duomo (cathedral), where Arima lived was the residence of charcoal burners. These were some of the city's poorest residents, along with prostitutes and general outcasts and lost souls of society. Their clothes and faces were dusted black from their work.

Arima had great skills with potions and spells, and she helped the poor locals of the neighbourhood with her healing herbs. When the Great Plague devastated the city's population around 1630, all the residents of Via

---

* *Strega* is the Italian for witch, after which a herbal Italian liqueur, dating from 1860, is named. I bought a bottle for research purposes! It is made with herbs and spices including mint, fennel and saffron. It is still made in Benevento, and there is a witch figure cast into the glass whilst its label depicts the *strega* dancing under the famous walnut tree that we heard of in Section One.

Laghetto survived, because Arima cast a spell over the area, protecting it. (People have since posed the more scientific explanation that it was the antibiotic properties of the charcoal that saved them. Perhaps it was a little of both...)

Other stories of Arima were that at night she organized parties and banquets, prepared potions, and danced on rooftops at the sabbaths before flying to the Piazza della Vetra. This was where executions were carried out for those who had been convicted of the most serious crimes, among which was witchcraft, and in 1641, it was here that the last two witches condemned in the city, were burned alive.

Any traces of Arima are lost: no document recorded her death, nor does her name appear among those condemned to the stake in Milan. I wonder if she was hidden or spirited away to safety by those she saved...

Kitchen Witch Celebrations for New Year

Some celebrate new year at Samhain, some at Hogmanay. Whenever and however you celebrate, bringing light to the darkest point of the year can be a comfort and joy, and, with the dormant season of the earth, a chance to pause and reflect. What paths and journeys have brought you here to this point? What gifts have you been blessed with over the year and festive season? Have you taken time to be truly grateful for the roof above your head and food on your plate? What are your wishes for the year ahead?

Celebrating Today

(Gather friends and family to welcome in the New Year. Light candles and fires for the occasion. Sing "Auld Lang Syne" together.

(Eat one grape for every strike of the clock at midnight (a tradition in Spain and Latin America).

(Open the front and back door of the home to let the New Year in and the old year out. (A tradition in British Isles and Europe and a favourite of my aunt, who kicks the doors as well just to make sure the years don't dawdle!)

☾ Plan a night out or celebration in with your fellow Kitchen Witches on January 6th.

IMBOLC

Imbolc, from the Gaelic word *oimelc/oimealg* which means "ewes milk," and *Imbolg,* meaning "in the belly," referencing pregnant livestock, February 1st or 2nd (dependent on the year), is the festival marking the first small signs of spring. Though it is not yet spring, the first signs of rebirth can be seen: the first flowers, buds and leaves. The days are lengthening, the birds begin to re-build their nests, and the dawn chorus begins. If you were part of an agricul-tural cycle, February is the month that you would begin preparing the land.

St Brigid's Day

In Ireland this time in early February is *Feile Brighde,* "the quickening of the year." This mid-point between the Winter Solstice and Spring Equinox, was personified for many Irish communities in the form of the goddess Brigid or St. Brigid (depending on your beliefs and culture, she is embodied in both goddess and Christian saint form). Brigid is the anglicized version of her name. You may come across many other different variants of her name includ-ing Brigit, Bridget, Brighde, Bride, Bridie, as is often the way with popular deities, they shift and morph as they travel through culture, times and stories.

Sweeping her green cloak across the land, Brigid revives the earth from its winter slumber. Offerings were made to entreat fertility and abundance, bonfires were set, hearths blazed, and candles were lit to offer Brigid and the season a warm welcome. Soda bread, apple cakes, barm brack and fresh but-ter, were served and savoured. Since the late 1500s, when the potato arrived in Ireland, it has been a staple food. A dish called colcannon made of mashed potato, cabbage and butter (sometimes with the addition of herbs, greens and spring onion) is now very much considered a traditional Imbolc dish.

As Brigid was thought to visit homes on the eve of her feast, food and drink would be laid out. Families may have a special meal, some of which would be set aside for Brigid's visit, to welcome her in with the hope she would bless the house for the coming year. Women might weave dolls of Brigid from wheat stalks or make Brigid's Crosses from reeds to hang in the house for luck and protection for the coming year. A little bed might also be made for the doll, or as a place for Brigid herself to rest – a tradition continued in many Irish and Scottish homes today. As the hearth is sacred to Brigid, one might "smoor" or smother the fire and rake the ashes smooth. And in the morning, if a mark could be seen in the ashes it was indication that Brigid has passed through.

Candlemas

To Christians, February 2nd is known as Candlemas. Also known as the Feast of the Purification of the Blessed Virgin Mary, and *Candelaria* in Spanish speaking countries. Like some other Christian festivals, Candlemas has foundations in pagan practice.

Candles would be taken to local churches to be blessed and then carried in procession, placed in windows and used through the year to literally and symbolically drive away the darkness and nurture the light.

Candlemas day used to be held in the old pagan times as a kind of saturnalia, with dances and torches and many unholy rites. But these gave occasion to so much ill conduct that in the ninth century the Pope abolished the festival and substituted for it the Feast of the Purification of the Blessed Virgin, when candles were lit in her honour. Hence the name of Candlemas.

Jane Francesca Agnes Wilde, *Ancient Legends, Mystic Charms and Superstitions of Ireland* (1887)

In some places Candlemas and Brigid celebrations combined, as we see with customs brought together here that are still observed today:

As Candlemas Day comes round, the mistress and servants of each family taking a sheaf of oats, dress it up in woman's apparel, and after putting it in a large basket, beside which a wooden club is placed, they cry three times, "Briid is come! Briid is welcome!" This they do just before going to bed, and as soon as they rise in the morning, they look among the ashes, expecting to see the impression of Briid's club there, which if they do, they reckon it a true presage of a good crop and prosperous year.

M. Martin, *Description of the Western Isles of Scotland* (1703)

Brigid's Foods

Many legends were absorbed into the story of St. Brigid, who blesses homes and creates countless "food miracles." We've already seen that St. Brigid turned water into ale back in the chapter about alewives. In her presence cows may give double their usual yield, dairy churnings are increased to fill many vessels with butter, one sack of malt makes eighteen vats of ale, and the bread supply is always sufficient for guests.

Brigid connects to the "cauldron of plenty," a common motif in Celtic literature and legend. And many of her legends could connect her to witch crafts. She was believed to be a healer and teacher of herbcraft, and many plants and flowers are thought to be sacred to her (including heather, chamomile, blackberries and rosemary). New greens and early spring herbs were also part of Brigid's feast including the first shoots of wild garlic, nettles, burdock, sorrel and dandelion. Dandelion is another plant potentially associated with Brigid, one of its names in Irish, *bior na bride,* Flame of Brigid, insinuates a possible connection to her sacred flame which is tended in Kildare.

For our ancestors, simple food magic or superstitions were an act of faith in blessings to come: fires create warmth, light increases light, golden rounds of cheese and butter bring on the sun and feasting begets more feasting! A cause for culinary celebration indeed!

Hearth Cakes, Bannock Cakes and Pancakes

> *Solmonath can be called the month of hearthcakes, which they used to offer to their gods in that month.*
>
> **Bede, *The Reckoning of Time* (725)**

February for the Anglo-Saxons was *Solmonath* – Cake Moon or Cake Month. Hearth cakes were cooked directly on the hearth stone or in the embers using the last grains from the autumn's harvest and were offered up to the gods. *Solmonath* can also mean mud or earth, and so it might be that this month is time to use up the very last of the earth's bounty, as one patiently watched to new signs of life in the dirt.

Anglo-Saxons called these small hearth cakes by the Old English term *cycel* – pronounced *kitchel* – meaning "to cook," and words drawn from this root include kitchen, cookies and cake.

Bannocks are a simple kind of oatcake that were baked in Scotland for pretty much every occasion, as oats are one of the few grains that grow well in the north of Scotland. The term "bannock" can be applied to any round cake baked or cooked from grain. They were often made as offerings to spirits, or used in divination. In one custom, they were rolled down hills: one side of the bannock was marked with a cross and the other a circle, if it landed cross side up, it meant life, circle side indicated death.

For "Bannock Night" a ring might be worked into the dough. The Bannock was shared out amongst the unmarried women and whoever got the piece with the ring would be the next married. Yule bannock was baked on Christmas morning as a gift for each person. Lughnasadh or Lammas bannock (on August 1st) might be made with the first grains of the first harvest. And Beltane bannock for summer was eaten on Beltane morning, to ensure health and abundance for your crops and herds.

Today in the British Isles it is pancakes we most associate with this time of year. Pancake Day or Shrove Tuesday can fall on any Tuesday between late February or early March dependant on the date of Easter. The custom of eating pancakes on Shrove Tuesday dates to the sixteenth century, as a way of using up the butter, eggs and sugar that would be given up during the Lenten season. In many parish churches, a popular Shrove Tuesday tradition is the ringing of the church bells (on this day, the toll is known as the Shriving Bell) described as a marker to both call to confession, or, for people to begin frying and tossing their pancakes and enjoying revels before the long fast of Lent.

The Russian Pancake Witch

In the week before Lent, Russians (and some Slavic neighbours like Belarus and Ukraine) may celebrate *Maslenitsa* (Pancake Week or Butter Week). A blend of a religious and folk holiday, it involves consuming many blinis (pancakes) and festivities such as dancing and winter sports. A full week of pancake feasting culminates by burning the straw effigy of a woman in traditional dress that gives her an air of the crone; this is Lady Maslenitsa, so she is the pancake lady or pancake witch, also thought of as the old witch of winter. She might be holding pancakes as she is burnt, and any remaining pancakes are thrown onto her pyre. Burning her is a symbolic farewell to winter, and farewell to pancakes for some time as Lent commences.

In France this celebration is known as *Mardi Gras* "Fat Tuesday," which is marked by feasting and costumed processions through the street. In Italy it is known as *Carnevale* (the root of our English word, carnival) – meaning "farewell to meat," and is held in the days before Ash Wednesday. Italians often wore masks and costumes to the *Carnevale* to disguise their identities whilst they frolicked, and still today families gather to dress up and celebrate in the streets.

The Kitchen Witch's Hedgerow and Garden

The quickening of the year brings the first beautiful blooms in soft milk tones of whites, yellows and creams: snowdrops, primroses, and daffodils. Sometimes they must make their way bravely through snowdrifts to bloom. The flowers of primrose – *Primula vulgaris* can be eaten raw, the leaves are better cooked as they can be tough.

Root vegetables and brassicas may still be in the vegetable garden: leeks, cabbages, kale and sprouts and herbs of rosemary and bay. And one may enjoy looking forward to the year ahead by sowing seeds indoors.

This is the time to enjoy pancakes with cream, milk and butter, particularly delicious on cold February days, enjoy with stewed apples and primrose flowers – golden treats that can brighten the grey skies we may see in February.

Kitchen Witch Celebrations for Imbolc

You may wish to plant both seeds and intentions at Imbolc. February is still winter, often cold, and grey, but within this time is a stirring, like seeds in the deep dark earth, a distant glimmer, a spark on the horizon. We can plant a seed at Imbolc, we can make our plans for the coming year, and with a little care and tending these seeds will grow through the growing light to ripen in the summer.

So think, perhaps, about intentions as you prepare to cross the threshold into a new burst of life. How can you nurture and nourish yourself for the journey? What seeds are you planting in your own life for the year ahead?

Celebrating Today

☾ Plant or tend snowdrops in your garden (or bring them in a pot into your kitchen). Often the first flowers of spring, their generic name Galanthus, is from the Greek *gala* (milk) and *anthos* (flower).

☾ Light a white candle with a small food offering, and perhaps weave a Brigid's Cross. An offering and invitation for Brigid to bless your home.

☾ Make colcannon or bannock cakes, perhaps with your own homemade butter (simply overwhip cream until the fats solidify and separate from the buttermilk).

☾ Make pancakes for breakfast…or dinner on Shrove Tuesday.

☾ Celebrate your own Cake Month. Bake your favourite cake and enjoy with loved ones.

SPRING EQUINOX AND OSTARA

The Spring or Vernal Equinox occurs each year in the Northern Hemisphere around March 20th-23rd and indicates the equal split of day and night. To many it signifies the beginning of spring. On this date, on the Wheel of the Year, we find the festival of Ostara.

Ostara – both the goddess figure and the festival name – is drawn from Germanic folklore. But we see many similar themes through other European cultures when it comes to the spring goddesses – almost always they are portrayed as young maidens. These are goddesses of light, full of the joy, promise and potential of the young year, very much an anthropomorphised form of the season of spring. Ancient Rome and Greece would have honoured deities like Flora, Persephone, Eos and Aurora through feasts and celebrations as well as variants of symbols of the season: eggs, rabbits, chicks and flowers – the bounty of the natural world at springtime.

When the monastic scholar Bede explored the Anglo-Saxon tradition, in his writing in *The Reckoning of Time,* he talks of this season as *Eosturmonath,* the month of Saxon goddess Ēostre. Called *Ostern* in German, the root of these names is "East," where the sun rises. Folklorist Jacob Grimm suggested Ostara as the Germanic version of Ēostre, and that's the name most commonly picked up for the Wheel of the Year with Ostara and Ēostre considered one and the same.

Eostra, the radiant creature of the Dawn. It will be remembered that it was the worship, not of Balder, but of Eostra, which the Christian missionaries found so deeply imbedded that they adopted her name and transferred it to Easter.[...]

Closely intertwined with Nature worship we find the later Christian rites and ceremonies. For the new teaching did not oust the old, and for many centuries the mind of the average man halted half-way between the two faiths. If he accepted Christ he did not cease to fear the great hierarchy of unseen powers of Nature, the worship of which was bred in his very bone. [...]

The ancient festivals of Yule and Eostra continued under another guise and polytheism still held its sway. The Devil became one with the gloomy and terrible in Nature, with the malignant elves and dwarfs. Even with the warfare between the beneficent powers of sun and the fertility of Nature and the malignant powers of winter, the Devil became associated. Nor did men cease to believe in the Wyrd, that dark, ultimate fate goddess who, though obscure, lies at the back of all Saxon belief. It was in vain that the Church preached against superstitions.

Eleanour Sinclair Rohde, *The Old English Herbals* (1922)

Easter

Whereas the Spring Equinox and Ostara are relatively set in their date, Easter in the Christian calendar can range from anywhere between March and April: it's a moveable feast. The date for Easter is plotted each year as the Sunday that follows the first full moon that occurs after the Spring Equinox. (I've always quite enjoyed this very pagan way to ascertain the date of a Christian holiday!)

Easter Foods

Eggs

Eggs have played a central role in spring rites and feasts for thousands of years. For their symbolism of rebirth and renewal, from ancient civilisations to modern Europe, eggs are sacred objects embodying the essence of life. Eggs embodied the fertilising vitality of the spring sun because it was when hens, cued by increasing light, began laying once again. So eggs were, and are, popular for decoration, gifts and offerings to people and deities alike. They are also a valuable protein source, especially after a long winter.

Decorated eggs might be coloured with dyes and painted with magical symbols or words. In Eastern Europe, these ritual eggs are today called *pysanka* or *pisankin* (from the root word "to write"). In the modern-day, we may see painted eggs, dyed eggs, chocolate eggs and eggs with gifts inside. Decorated eggs may well be found being rolled down grassy hills in England, amongst other merriment of pace- or peace-eggers, who, like the mummers of midwinter, dress fantastically and perform plays and songs door-to-door, seeking offerings from households of eggs and foods. You can still find a few pace-egg players and plays in the north of England.

Simnel Cake

Simnel cake is a fruitcake often topped with marzipan and spring flowers, traditionally eaten through the British Isles for Mothering Sunday[*] and Easter Sunday. Mothering Sunday is a Christian holiday celebrated on the fourth Sunday of Lent by many denominations across Europe. Servants were given the day off and visited their families, home and "mother church." It was also a reprieve from the fasting of Lent, so various types of cakes have long been part of Mothering Sunday fun, especially a nice high-calorie simnel cake, as a gift to one's parents.

Not far from me in Wiltshire, the town of Devizes have their very own style of the simnel cake. The Devizes star simnel is made with currants and lemon peel, coloured golden with saffron and always made in a star shape, then boiled, baked and glazed. In contrast, the Bury simnel cake is made with the addition of nuts and cinnamon (and in some recipes with cherries and marzipan icing).

Crossed Buns

On Good Friday, it is a custom in England to eat hot cross buns, sweet bread rolls made with raisins and dried citrus peel, lightly spiced with cinnamon, nutmeg and cloves and topped with the sign of the holy cross. In folklore, the cross upon the bun meant it could be hung from ceilings as a warding device, similarly cutting a cross in the dough of any loaf of bread was useful in stopping the Devil sitting on it and preventing it from rising. In Ireland a cross is cut in the top of a loaf of soda bread before baking to "let the fairies out."

---

[*] Although in Britain Mothering Sunday is often also called Mothers' Day, it's not connected with the American festival of the same name, which is why they are celebrated on different days: America, Canada, New Zealand and Australia all celebrate Mother's Day in May.

The Easter Witch

Just as with La Bafana in Italy, not all witches in folklore are portrayed as bad; some are connected to joyful folklore traditions (but like many, they may have a dark past). In Sweden and Finland, it is an Easter tradition for children to dress as *paskkarringar* – Easter witches. They dress up as little hag figures, wearing headscarves, and with rosy cheeks painted on their faces. These little old folks carry copper kettles and cauldrons to hold their bounty, as they go door-to-door wishing people a happy Easter and receiving sweets in return. They may also use their birch and feather brooms to sweep away bad luck.

The tradition is based around folklore that before Easter, witches would fly to the Island of Blakulla[†] to feast and dance with the Devil, who held his earthly parties in meadows on this island during the Witches' Sabbath. As the witches were on their flight back from their revels, Swedes would light fires to scare them away, a practice honoured today by the bonfires and fireworks across the land in the days leading up to Easter Sunday.

The *paskkarring* tradition has been around since at least the early nineteenth century, though originally it was teenagers and young adults who dressed up to cause mischief, like guisers in England. Like many traditions before it, the act of warding against witches and casting out evils has become to some, a celebration of witches, and to others, a chance for revelry and games.

Witchy traditions in Sweden include both the cheerful Easter Witches welcoming in the springtide and that household poppet figure we met earlier: The Kitchen Witch. In Sweden, at least in modern times, it seems the witch is a favourable symbol, and to have a witch in your house brings good luck and blessings.

The Kitchen Witch's Hedgerow and Garden

Birch twigs begin to bud with catkins under blue skies. Herbs and flowers grow with the scent and colour of mint and violets; hope is in the air. But from March into April, the winter crops of cabbage and kale from Imbolc and the

---

† Blakulla is a real island in the Baltic Sea, but it is referred to most often now as Blå Jungfrun, The Blue Maiden, because sea-lore suggests that saying the island's real name whilst at sea would brew up a storm.

stores of potatoes, apples, and roots veg might be running low, and with spring vegetables only just sown this time was sometimes known as the 'hungry gap,' a time when the 'need foods' of hedgerows would have been particularly valuable.

Early spring is peak nettle season; pick tender top leaves (with gloves) and use in teas and soups. Wild garlic springs up in fresh greens and whites, scenting woodlands. It's easily identifiable by that intense scent and can be mixed with butter or used in place of basil for pesto.

Come April, the spring sun shines on golden treasures; bees are producing honey and the hens will be laying their precious eggs.

Kitchen Witch Celebrations for Ostara

The Spring Equinox is a celebration of expanding energy and warmth, like the rising sun in the east, this is a new dawn on a new season. Every day after today will be longer than the night, reason for hope to rise as well! It's time to step out of the hungry gap, the dark winter, and the cold, and into the light.

Celebrating Today

☾ Grab your broom and duster and spring clean your home.

☾ Bring spring in…pick or buy a posy of spring flowers for your kitchen table: tulips, daffodils, hyacinth, fresh beech leaves…

☾ Crystalise primroses and violets by painting with egg white and sprinkling with sugar – a fabulous way to decorate spring cakes; beautiful and edible.

☾ The first chocolate eggs were made for easter in Europe in the early nineteenth century. Enjoy bringing the magic of chocolate and the egg symbol together in this sweet treat by buying or making your own.

☾ Explore recipes from your local area: do you have a local simnel cake recipe like in Devizes? Or an Easter treat unique to your family?

☾ Dye boiled eggs with natural dye. Try onion skins for yellow, red cabbage for blue, turmeric for orange, beetroot for pink and spinach for green. You can draw patterns on them first with a white wax crayon.

☾ Oh, and don't crush those eggshells, you never know when a witch might need one to set sail in!

BELTANE

In Celtic traditions, the spelling of this May festival is Bealtaine and directly translates as "mouth of fire," coming from the Irish Gaelic *béal* (mouth) and *tine* (fire). This is the opening to the summer season and fire is its most important element. If splitting the year simply into summer and winter, we are tipping into summer, so a fine thing to celebrate! This might have been a marker for nomadic farmers to take their livestock to summer pastures, potentially to return come Samhain.

Beltane is considered the anglicized version of Bealtaine (and is the spelling I've used in my Wheel of the Year diagram). This version also introduces differing ideas about the meaning of the word – becoming now "bright fires" or "good fires" and a possible connection to the Celtic sun god Bel/Belanus/Baal. Direct connection can't always be drawn between deities and festivals via historical texts, however, at festival times that celebrate sunshine and light, it seems very likely that regional deities would have been connected to the celebration, for those who considered them patrons or who sought favour. Beltane is the celebration of light, fertility, and the coming of summer, and so it seems right that Bel may well oversee things.

This gateway into summer is hailed with joy, and the day recognised as the first of the season is naturally one of the most important days in the calendar and a time for potential magic. Traditional Gaelic/Celtic festivities are still celebrated in Ireland, Scotland, Cornwall, the Isle of Man, Wales with variants of name, and May Day festivities run all through Europe.

Fire and Flowers

The sacred fires of Beltane would have been particularly important for areas that relied heavily on livestock. Ancient Celtic tribes used to bring their cattle out of the winter barns at Beltane and drive them between two huge balefires for purification and protection before they were released into the summer pastures as a symbolic safeguard and blessing. These May fires also provided light and blessing for homes, as all the fires in the area may be rekindled from these sacred flames. Each townsperson would take home fire to kindle their own, a practice often repeated at Beltane's opposite on the Wheel, Samhain.

More arable areas would have focused more on garlands of flowers and greenery, to encourage crops to prosper. Rituals throughout Europe included a May Queen, a young maiden crowned with garlands, who may have represented the embodiment of spring, or spring goddesses like Flora, a Roman fertility goddess of flowers and springtime.

The maypole – a tall pole, crowned with flowers and hung with ribbons – would be danced around on May Day (a tradition still popular in areas of England, Germany and Austria) and English folkloric figures like Jack in the Green or The Green Man may need to be killed or paraded to release the spirit of summer.

Caudle

People in the north of Scotland cut a trench in the ground; they then kindled a fire and dressed a repast of milk and eggs, something like a custard. This being done, they kneaded a cake of oatmeal, and toasted it before the fire. The custard was then eaten, and the cake was broken into pieces and thrown into a bag, not, however, before one of the pieces was burned black. Every one of the company in turn was blindfolded, and drew out a piece of the cake; and he who drew out the burned piece was dedicated to Baal, in order to render the year fruitful. The person supposed to be devoted was then compelled to leap three times over the fire, as symbolical of the sacrifices offered to this god in former ages.

James Grant, *The Mysteries of All Nations/Strange Customs Fables and Tales* (1880)

This account is very similar to the Anglo-Saxon *aecer-bot* charm, which can be found in texts dated to pre-1200, a field remedy for infertile land. Before dawn, the farmer takes chunks of turf from all four corners of their land and pours over them milk, oil and honey, with little bits of the plants of the land before covering again with the turf, speaking an invocation to Mother Earth.

This custardy mix mentioned was often called caudle, made from eggs, milk, butter, grain and, possibly, alcohol.

These resources offered to the land would have been very precious foodstuffs – even more so if crops were not forthcoming. So, there was a real sacrifice to giving them to the land, but with that, a respect for the land and the crops was bestowed. A good harvest was not considered something they were entitled to, but a gift from Mother Earth.

Walpurgisnacht

In Germany, May Eve is *Walpurgisnacht,* the night of the mass flight of witches to the high peaks of mountaintops to dance and make magic and see in the arrival of spring – it is also known as *Hexennacht,* Witches' Night. Over much of Europe, the eve of May, like all the seasonal gateway festivals is when witches and otherworldly beings were thought to be out, about and causing trouble. The Brocken is the highest peak of the Harz mountain range (and the highest peak of Northern Germany), this is the spot where witches and devilish beings were thought to gather on *Walpurgisnacht.*

On *Walpurgisnacht,* one might hear clanging pots, chanting, singing, shooting into the air, and see bonfires which would be jumped through and danced around (both townsfolk and witches were said to do this – rituals seem to vary from warding off witches to celebrations inspired by them) and while bonfires might still be lit to scare away witches and burn effigies, modern-day celebrations are just as likely to welcome the witches and their dancing night!

Among the lore of the Harz mountains and *Walpurgisnacht* is that of a plateau within the mountain range called the *"Hexentanzplatz,"* which means "the Witches Dance Floor." According to German folklore, the coming of the warm season was marked by seasonal goddesses and witches dancing away the snow for the growth of spring and summer.

> *The Witches' excursion takes place on the first night in May...they ride up Blocksberg on the first of May, and in 12 days must dance the snow away; then Spring begins... Here they appear as elflike, godlike maids.*

Jacob Grimm, *Deutsche Mythologie* **(1835)**

People congregated, danced, and had all manner of festivities in the mountains to celebrate the changing of the seasons. Connected goddesses include Holda, who we met in the Yule section, who often held company with witches and the mountain forest goddesses. The *Hexentanzplatz* and the Brocken mountain peak were Old Saxon sites of worship, at which pagan celebrations were held. We know at least part of this story is true, as excavations have found an altar used to sacrifice animals on the mountain top.

> *The witches invariably resort to places where formerly justice was administered, or sacrifices were offered [...] under the lime, under the oak, at the pear tree [...] sometimes they dance at the place of execution, under the gallows-tree [...] The fame of particular witch-mountains extends over wide kingdoms, in*

the same way as high mountains are named after gods. [...] Almost all the
witch-mountains were once hills of sacrifice, boundary-hills, or salt-hills.

Jacob Grimm, *Deutsche Mythologie* (1835)

According to legend, dancing at the *Hexentanzplatz* was banned by invading Christian Franks. But on May Eve night, when King Charlemagne ordered his soldiers to guard the place to ensure no pagan revels occurred, the pagan Saxons dressed up as story-book witches, complete with pointed hats and broomsticks in hand, and chased the Frankish guards away with their cackles and cries. Which I really hope is true... If you are going to be demonised, you may as well use that fear to clear your dancefloor, right?!

St. Walpurga

We've already seen how the Church may combine festivities with pagan roots. Stories and celebrations are layered over and over each other, a layer cake of customs and celebrations.

St. Walpurga/Walburga, for whom *Walpurgisnacht* is named, was, interestingly enough, a wise woman and healer hailed for curing ailments and warding against witchcraft. So, some healing women did escape persecution. The Church's protection would have helped hugely, as all her skills were considered gifts from God. She died around 777 CE and she was canonised on May 1st, which became the Feast of St. Walpurga. The eve of this feast, *Walpurgisnacht*, was already known as a *Hexennacht* (Witches' Night). We are familiar with Christian festivities being laid over older pagan ones, and perhaps Walpurga's presence was considered shrewd on this night as useful for protection from those merry witches.

Or perhaps she was used to replace earlier pagan deities. The earliest representation of Walpurga is in the eleventh-century *Hitda Codex*; Hitda was abbess of a women's monastery in Meschede, Germany. And she commissioned the work, on the dedication page Hitda herself is depicted presenting the codex to St. Walpurga, the patron saint of Meschede.

St. Walpurga holds a golden stalk of grain, which could well be drawn from imagery of a Grain Mother or Earth Goddess. Or it may be from her own folklore; miracles credited to the saint include: saving a child from starving with three ears of wheat; calming rabid dogs; healing the sick; and helping women in childbirth. Rural folks fashioned corn dollies, much as we do around the British Isles for goddesses like Brigid, and would seek St. Walpurga's blessing of their grain. In statues and paintings, you'll also see her holding books and little potion bottles for her healing oil in reference to her wisdom and healing. Today, where she is still remembered, she is patroness against storms, diseases, famine and watches over farmers and their harvests.

For some, Beltane and the Witches' Night became a feast day for St. Walpurga, but many customs remain relatively unchanged: dancing and leaping in and around fires is a staple of the night's customs, before and after the saintly name change. And folks still practised simple sympathetic magic, hoping that grain would grow as high as the farmer could jump on *Walpurgisnacht*. Misfortunes were symbolically burned on the fires. Straw figures were made to represent things like illness, disease, and bad luck, and these, along with remnants of the last year were burnt in the hope of a brighter year to come.

The Kitchen Witch's Hedgerow and Garden

As May turns to June and summer arrives, gooseberries ripen, sprays of creamy white elderflowers bloom, and sorrel also begins to appear: a herbaceous plant, its medicinal properties (reducing inflammation) and citrusy flavour have made it a favourite for foragers.

Sweet woodruff is a wild plant native to much of Europe. Emerging in early spring, its leaves arranged in a star shape, followed by tiny white flowers in May. Sweet woodruff has a connection to witches as, firstly, it blooms in May, so it's often used in Walpurgisnacht celebrations and warding off evil spirits, and also for its medicinal value. A herbal cure for pain and inflammation, sweet woodruff is said to soothe weariness of the feet and joints in travellers, which is entirely appropriate to this celebration, as witches were thought to travel far and wide for their mountain revelries, to gather just before midnight at crossroads, mountain tops, and in forests.

May Wine is a favourite for Beltane. Like wassail, the contents can vary greatly, and it's the social elements that make it a ritual. Alcoholic versions use honey mead or white wine as the base, and honey and herbs in season like sweet woodruff, strawberries, and other herbs and fruits may be added for flavour. In celebrations in Germany, May Wine (known as *Maibowle*) is made by steeping the leaves of sweet woodruff in white wine and sweetening it with sugar. Other uses for sweet woodruff flowers would be for headdresses and altar flowers, as their sweet scent were thought to protect against malevolent spirits and bad luck.

Headdresses and flowers festooning altars would also have been found in the ancient Roman celebration of *Floralia,* the festival held in honour of the goddess Flora, the goddess of blossoming plants, held in Roman cities from the end of April and into May. This was a celebration of flowers and the promise of them becoming fruit later in the year.

Kitchen Witch Celebrations for Beltane

Beltane is a time of growth, of movement and blooming. A time perhaps to connect to your primal spirit and move, dance, play in nature, and leap over fires! Listen deeply to rhythms and inspiration that arise. Well past the equinox, we are closer now to midsummer than midwinter. The light of spring and summer dances in. Allow yourself to unfurl like a flower bud: have a good stretch and reawaken! This is a time for growth and fertility in all things in your life from creating new relationships and ideas to new projects and adventures.

Celebrating Today

☾ Buy or harvest gooseberries. I enjoy them raw, crisp and sour as hell. But you can also stew them with sugar and mix with cream for a gooseberry fool.

☾ If you fear evil spirits on May Eve, lay the spiky branches of the gooseberry bush by your doorway for protection.

☾ Gather flowers or greenery from your garden or mindfully from nature, and create a garland or posy for your kitchen. Or make a flower crown or floral wreath.

☾ Enjoy a cold glass of wine in the sun. (You may feel inspired to create May Wine with seasonal herbs and flowers, or simply uncork a bottle!)

☾ Collect elderflower blossoms, and make them into champagne, it takes a few weeks to ferment so you'll have a refreshing drink in good time to raise a glass for midsummer.

☾ Dance! You might want to make a maypole to dance around with friends and family, but the kitchen floor can also be a very fine *Hexentanzplatz.*

☾ If you have the space, build a bonfire.

SUMMER SOLSTICE, MIDSUMMER AND LITHA

As we move through the Wheel of the Year and to June, we arrive at the counterpoint to Yule and Winter Solstice: the Summer Solstice, also called Litha. Like in winter, for a few days, the sun appears to rise and set in exactly the same place: "solstice" means "sun standing still." It has, for thousands of years, been considered a sacred and magical time, a celestial pause.

In these warmer times, there is sense of revelry, of flower fairies and forest sprites dancing in the sunbeams. There is a sense that magic can be found: knowledge of the land, the fae, their secrets and their ability to cross between worlds. The fire festival of midsummer, along with the great fires lit, along with more light and warmth from the sun, give the sense of a great lighting up of hidden places and mysteries.

Summer Solstice and Midsummer

The festivities associated with the peak of summer cluster around a few dates in England and Europe. While the event of Summer Solstice occurs between June 20th and 23rd, Midsummer's Day is fixed in European calendars as June 24th. It is also known as St. John's Day or the Feast of St. John the Baptist, in a classic pagan-rooted, saint-overlapped combination we are now pretty familiar with.

Midsummer was a popular festival throughout England for centuries. Rural communities marked it with Morris dancing, parades, drinking and feasting, blessing of crops and the ritual exile of fiendish spirits. Midsummer's Day is still a very popular festival in Sweden, Latvia and Lithuania, where the Midsummer festival, or its eve, are public holidays. The exact dates today vary among different cultures, countries and customs but is primarily held close to the Summer Solstice.

Litha

Summer Solstice is also known as Litha, an Anglo-Saxon name for summer used in the Anglo-Saxon calendar for the Summer Solstice itself as well as for the months of June and July. June is 'before Litha' or first summer month, July is 'after Litha' or second summer month. Now it has been given a new lease of life as it features in the Wheel of the Year, again, this is a modern addition in this layout of the Wheel, but based in historical usage.

The little we know of Litha is found by works like that of Bede, who wrote that "Litha means 'gentle' or 'navigable,' because in both those months the calm breezes are gentle and they were wont to sail upon the smooth sea."[21]

Summer Solstice is the longest day of the year, and from here the days become shorter once again. Seeing in the sunrise on this special day is a favoured pastime by pagans old and new. Besides feasts and fires, rituals might include the seeking of protection from unseen forces. Sun wheels were woven from stalks and various rituals performed for protection throughout the longest day of the year and especially so if one were married on this day. Marriages and hand-fasting rituals were common in summer, and people may be married on Litha as part of the celebration.

Becoming a Witch

In Cornwall, some say that witches gathered on the eve of Midsummer near Zennor (home of the mermaids) to feast around a bonfire. They would gather at standing stones, flying in on ragwort stems.

In Cornish lore, anyone may become a witch at midsummer, if so desired. All you need do is put bread into the mouth of a toad, who will swallow the bread and then breathe on you three times. Touching designated "witches stones" at special times like midsummer is also said to have the effect of turning one into a witch.

A similar connection to bread and witches can be found in *Household Tales with other Traditional Remains* by Sidney Oldall Addy (1895):

Witchcraft may be acquired in the following way: When taking sacrament at church, instead of eating the cake which the parson gives you, save it, and wait until all the people have gone home. Then walk backwards round the church nine times, looking into every window and door as you go. Then return home, and, as you go, give the cake to the first living thing that you meet, be it dog, cat, or any other animal.

Burning Witches at Midsummer

For the most part, today in Europe, at least, witch hunts have ended, and witches are no longer burned. But the mythology of witch persecution is embedded in European culture, and the burning of witches in the form of effigies, especially on pagan holidays, still happens.

In Denmark and some parts of England, effigies of witches made of rags and straw are burnt on midsummer bonfires. In many places bonfires were used, among other things, to scare away witches and evil spirits for the rest of the year. When black smoke begins to rise from the flames, a cheer goes up and drinks are raised: this is a symbol of the witch flying away. On Beltane on the Isle of Man, islanders set fire to the gorse, sacred to the Cailleach, crone goddess of winter, to burn out the witches thought to gather there in the form of hares.

The Kitchen Witch's Hedgerow and Garden

Hedges and gardens are at their lushest and most spectacular in June; everything is blooming, especially fragrant roses, wild and cultivated. Meadowsweet, wild strawberries, foxgloves...all burst in colour in the hedgerows, and bees buzz and hum as they feast on nectar and pollen-rich blooms. This time of year offers a wealth of wild treats: yarrow leaves and borage, with its blue, star-shaped flowers, can be slipped into cool drinks and iced teas. And one could brew beer with harvested heather and gorse, which grow along our British coastlines and are particularly abundant now.

Ragwort is found in fields and wild places. It can rise three or four feet high with yellow flowers. This is what the Cornish witches fly on. It might be the height of the stems, the fact that they grow in wild spaces and the fact that they flower in June and July that seemed to connect ragwort to witches and the fae. According to *Culpeper's Complete Herbal,* ragwort is under the command of Venus and cleanses and heals, which seems appropriate for a witch.

Honey from the bees we wassailed in midwinter may now be ready to collect. And in gardens and farms, we will be seeing juicy berries and fruits such as raspberries and strawberries ripening ready to eat – their wonderful red fruits reflecting the heat and warmth of the season. There is something particularly magical and joyful about storing the sun's energy at Litha within jams, pies and puddings.

The early mornings are light and bright and steeped with the jubilant dawn chorus of robins, blackbirds, woodpigeons, wrens and warblers. This midsummer period is also the perfect time to gather and dry medicinal herbs for the year. Many believed that witches adopted the same practice of gathering ingredients for their potions at midsummer and would meet up afterwards for their seasonal celebrations.

Kitchen Witch Celebrations for Midsummer

Here at the solstice, there is a pause in the sun's journey in the eyes of the ancient people of the British Isles. This sacred pause was celebrated and honoured with great circles of stone and wood where people have for generations gathered to watch the sun rise. They lit bonfires on hills, decorated holy wells with blossoms, and burnt herbs to bless animals, homes and farms.

Summer is, as you may imagine, connected to the element of fire, and the energy of rising, joy, and heat. You can connect to this energy in many ways. Walk barefoot on warm grass. Swim in a sparkling river or the sea. Take your cue from the solstice sun and pause, be still. Stand and be where you are, with the season: feel the light and warmth. Listen to the buzz and hum of the bees, the chirp of birdsong and flap of wings, watch the dance of the butterfly through tall grasses, breathe in the scents of lavender, rose, and honeysuckle, the multisensory song of summer is here, resplendent in the bright light of the sunbeams. Listen. Breathe. And smile.

We are already at the turning point; every day after this, a little shorter, and winter will, in time, begin to beckon us from the distant wilds, but not yet, my friend, not yet!

Celebrating Today

(Go fruit picking and enjoy an afternoon of making jam from the first strawberries and raspberries of the season (both start fruiting around June)

(Feed some toads (though I cannot guarantee this will make you a witch!) They prefer mealworms to bread. If you have a pond in your garden, consider creating wood or stone piles to offer toads refuge.

(Take a moment to stand still in your kitchen, and light a candle for all witches accused, ostracised, tortured or killed.

(Pick or buy a bunch of beautiful June roses; perhaps make rose water, rose petal jam or crystalise a few petals to decorate cakes.

(Rise with the dawn or stay up late till the last light to welcome in the solstice.

(Gather bunches of herbs and hang them up to dry for cooking or burning in the months ahead.

(Seek out standing stones, stone circles, monoliths, or any stone, tree, or mountain that is sacred for you, for your own solstice ritual.

LAMMAS AND LUGHNASADH

Falling on August 1st, this is the first of three harvest festivals on the Wheel of the Year: Lughnasadh, Autumn Equinox and Samhain. They cover several months due to different crops ripening at different times. Lughnasadh, also called Lammas, is the first harvest festival marking the beginning of the harvest season and also the eventual weakening of the sun's light and heat.

Lammas

Lammas is the festival of the wheat and grain harvest, the name comes from the Anglo-Saxon hlaf-mas and Old English *hlafmæsse/ hlammæsse*, meaning "loaf mass" or "loaf feast". For early Christians and in the Anglo-Saxon tradition, Lammas is the festival of the 'first fruits' of the harvest season. It was a time to give thanks for the beginning of the harvest season and to entreat deities to guard over the still-ripening crops that remained.

> *When we take corns at Lammas, we take but about two sheaves, when the corns are full; or two stalks of kail, or thereby, and that gives us the fruit of the corn-land or kail-yard, where they grew. And it may be, we will keep it until Yule or Pasche (Easter), and then divide it amongst us.*

From Isobel Gowdie's witch trial testimony (1662)

Bringing in the harvest was a communal act, so whatever the religious or cultural inclinations, harvest is a great 'bringer-together-er'!

The main Lammas custom during the Middle Ages to honour the harvest was baking bread and cakes of the freshly harvested crop. Bread made from the first gathered grains might then be broken into four pieces and placed at the four corners of a barn, home, or field to ensure protection and prosperity. It was popular to form Lammas bread into the shape of a sheaf of corn, a custom that continues in some communities. The bread baked might be brought to the church for blessing. Leftover stalks might be made into corn dollies and poppets for blessing and protection.

Like many of these festivals, while observation has generally declined with the lessening importance of the agricultural year, many customs associated with Lammas/Lughnasadh are still celebrated in rural communities. Festivities can include feasting, sports, harvest festivals, and agricultural fairs.

Lughnasadh

Lughnasadh/Lughnasa is the Gaelic name for this first festival of harvest and it is celebrated throughout Ireland and some parts of Scotland and the Isle of Man. Named for the god Lugh, drawn from Irish mythology, Lugh is, to some, a deity of light and the sun, to others he is more closely connected with skill, battle, craft and wisdom.

Lughnasadh means "Lugh's gathering/assembly," and in some stories the god Lugh holds a funeral feast, rituals and games upon a hill-top in commemoration of his mother figure, Tailtiu, an earth goddess who died of exhaustion clearing the earth of Ireland for agriculture (in other versions she represented the dying vegetation that fed mankind.) Lughnasadh marks the passing of the seasons from summer into autumn in the Irish calendar – although, for many of us, August 1st is still very firmly in summertime.

A solemn cutting of the first corn of which an offering would be made to the deity by bringing it up to a high place and burying it; a meal of the new food and of bilberries of which everyone must partake; a sacrifice of a sacred bull, a feast of its flesh…a ritual dance-play perhaps telling of a struggle for a goddess and a ritual fight; an installation of a head on top of the hill and a triumphing over it by an actor impersonating Lugh.

Maire MacNeill, *The Festival of Lughnasa* (1962)

There was much eating, drinking, dancing, matchmaking, folk music and games, as well as athletic and sporting contests such as weight-throwing and the Gaelic sport of hurling.

Old texts tell of feasts and mythical funeral rites, both celebrations of the harvest and mourning of the coming end of summer.

"No man will travel this country," she said, *"who hasn't gone sleepless from Samhain, when the summer goes to its rest, until Imbolc, when the ewes are milked at spring's beginning, from Imbolc to Beltane at the summer's beginning and from Beltane to Brón Trogain,* earth's sorrowing autumn.*"*

Tochmarc Emire, tenth/eleventh century Irish text

The above passage comes from a collection of Irish tales *Tochmarc Emire* ("The Wooing of Emer"), during which Emer provides the earliest reference to the Irish pagan festivals that marked the changing of the seasons. It was celebrated more recently in Brian Friel's acclaimed play *Dancing at Lughnasa* (1990), set in Donegal in 1936 during the festival of Lughnasa.

Bilberry Magic

The bilberry, a member of the blueberry family, also known as whortle-berries, whinberries, huckleberries, blaeberries, fraughans and black-hearts, is native to Europe, namely the British Isles. They ripen at the end of July, perfect for harvest festivities around August 1st and are popular baked into pies and tarts, made into wine and eaten with cream for good luck (and probably to sweeten them as well).

The people in Cheshire do eate the blacke whortles in creame and milk, as in these southern parts we eate strawberries.

John Gerard, *The Herball* (1597)

In Ireland and Scotland, you may well head out on Bilberry Sunday (known as Fraughan Sunday in Ireland), a Sunday close to Lughnasadh, to gather berries, but this was also a chance to gather a spouse as well! Seeking berries on a sunny day could take many hours, and young men and women might enjoy this chance to socialise in fine weather. Bilberry Sunday became known as a time for courting, and girls might bake a bilberry pie to present to someone special to state their intentions.

Bilberries have long been used in medicine and cooking. They contain tannins and the dried fruit and leaves are still used to make some herbal medicines to reduce inflammation and lower blood pressure.

---

* In later sources *Brón Trogain* is known by the name *Lúgnasad*.

The Kitchen Witch's Hedgerow and Garden

In the evening sunlight of long summer days, fields shine golden, and baskets of mushrooms might be gathered, seen in fairy rings that appear overnight. You might just find the first apples of the season, and gardens may hold ripening tomatoes, courgettes, beans and peas. In farmers' fields, the first grain is harvested, and the first loaves made with it might be blessed for good luck.

The Kitchen Witch might have her mason jars ready, sitting in rows, clean and sparkling, waiting to hold the colours and flavours of July and August: juicy, bright and sweet cherries, redcurrants, bilberries, plums and raspberries.

Kitchen Witch Celebrations for Lammas and Lughnasadh

Many modern pagans mix the traditions of Lughnasadh and Lammas and similar harvest festivals from across Europe. The underlying theme of abundance and gratitude, bread and sunshine run through all these festivals, and then celebrations take form around these foundations: viewing human life as part of, not separate from, the natural world and giving thanks for the agricultural prosperity that sustains our common life every year.

If perhaps you harvest from your own garden, allotment, or the hedgerows, in the long evening light, take pause and reflect on the idea of the harvest. Have you planted other seeds, of intention this year in your life? Laid foundation for a new plan or a big decision? What is abundant and what are you grateful for?

Celebrating today

☽ Gather berries and make them into jams or muffins for a special breakfast feast.

☽ Bake a harvest loaf of bread. And break it with good company.

☽ Follow Lugh's lead and create your own joyful gathering – a picnic on a hillside, a barbecue or garden party perhaps!

☽ Seek fairy rings of mushrooms in forests and woodlands as they are most common in late summer to early autumn, after wet weather.

Mabon and Autumn Equinox

September 20th-23rd is the Autumn Equinox, where day and night are of equal length. There is still light, although the nights are getting steadily longer. As an equinox, this day would have been acknowledged in ancient cultures, but there is not so much evidence that our ancestors got quite so excited about this equinox as say Samhain and Yule, possibly because ahead of them lay a good period of hard work until the official end of the harvest at Samhain, and the revels of Yule and Christmas were not yet in sight. But we are now blessed with a choice to celebrate and revel in this festival if we wish.

Mabon (Wiccan), Harvest Home (rural English) or Alban Elfed (modern Druidic) is a time of thanksgiving and of sharing offerings to secure the blessings of deities during the coming winter months.

Activities at this time may include cider pressing, dancing and feasting (of course!) and the crowning of a Harvest King and Queen. Feasting would include the foods recently harvested in the local area: grains, nuts, apples, grapes and berries. Just as the first sheaves of corn were honoured at Lammas, in September the last sheaf was also significant. Practices with it varied widely, it might be brought into the house or barn where the Harvest Home feast was to be held, or burned and ground into ash, thought to be curative, or into a figure, known by names such as the "Kern Baby", "Corn Dolly" or "Harvest Queen", connected perhaps to pagan echoes of corn spirits or the Corn Mother.

In agricultural communities, one might be given the honoured title of Lord of the Harvest, a counterpart of a similar role at first harvest at Lammas, now it is to bring in the last sheaf of corn and declare the harvest safely gathered in before the harvest feasts could begin.

The Spirit of the Harvest
Look for hares in the fields on your next evening walk. In English folklore, the spirit of the harvested field was often depicted as a hare, as hares are often last to leave the harvested fields (the deer, pheasants, and foxes having long since fled to seek better hiding spots). Some say the hare is the goddess Ceres, or the *genius loci,* the protective spirit of a place.

When the hares depart the fields, they represent the spirit of life escaping as the last sheaf is cut. The last sheaf harvested is sometimes called "The Hare" and to cut it is to conclude the harvest. Poppets or charms made from this last-cut corn may be hung in homes or stables to offer protection from 'fairy raids,' witches and other malefic spirits.

> *On the last night of the year they [fairies] are kept out by decorating the house with holly; and the last handful of corn reaped should be dressed up as a Harvest Maiden (Maighdean Bhuan), and hung up in the farmer's house to aid in keeping them out till next harvest.* [22]

Mabon

The name of this festival time in the modern pagan/ Wiccan tradition as Mabon is credited to American Wiccan Aidan Kelly, as a reference to a character from Welsh mythology.

> *Back in 1974, I was putting together a "Pagan-Craft" Calendar... We have Gaelic names for the four Celtic holidays. It offended my aesthetic sensibilities that there seemed to be no Pagan names from the summer solstice or the fall equinox equivalent to Yule or Beltane – so I decided to supply them.*

Aidan Kelly, Patheos.com (2017)

He's also credited with drawing the names Ostara and Litha from folk practices, history and myth for use in the Wiccan wheel around the 1970s. (Interestingly that's one Welsh (Mabon); one Germanic (Ostara) and one Anglo-Saxon (Litha) name, which, along with the Germanic/Scandinavian Yule, make a decent mix of some of the myriad cultures that make up the British Isles.)

The name of Celtic god Mabon, was selected by Kelly for its connection to a more well-known motif of the story of Persephone and Demeter from ancient Greece, but many ancient civilisations have a story involving a deity who goes down into the Underworld or Otherworld and later returns to bring light and prosperity, and a figure of a 'child of light.'

In Welsh folklore Mabon is that being of light, being the son of Modron, the Great Goddess of the Earth, who was kidnapped three days after his birth.

Some pagans and Wiccans prefer simply to call these more recently named festivals equinoxes and solstices as Valiente and Gardner did, but at the very least it offers some interesting ideas in story and ongoing changes in cultures and folklore. It's not so very different from our widely used Gregorian calendar in present day, which was introduced by a Catholic pope, with months named after Roman gods, and week names after Norse gods and celestial bodies.

Mabon's Story

This is a short version of the tale of Mabon, which can be found in full in the collection of stories and myth: The Mabinogion *(written around the twelfth or thirteenth century and translated into English by Lady Charlotte Guest in 1848). Like the tale of Kerridwen and her cauldron, it features the relationship of mother and son and many fine animals.*

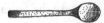

Once, a long time ago, there was a mother, Modron, which means Great Mother; she was beautiful and strong. Modron had a son whose name was Mabon, and he shone with light. But Mabon was stolen away into the darkness, and when Modron mourned, her tears swelled and flowed like a great ocean. Her world and the whole world fell into darkness without Mabon.

One day, a king arrived seeking to find Mabon. King Arthur and his knights had been set a task to hunt the mighty boar, one so strong and so fast that no hunter could track him down and kill him, save for the greatest huntsman of all. Folk whispered that if Mabon still lived and could be found, surely he could kill the boar. And so, King Arthur and his knights searched out the Blackbird, an old creature who had long guarded the gateway on the edge of dawn at the daylight gate.

"Blackbird," Arthur called, "We are looking for Mabon, who was stolen from his mother's side three nights after his birth. Do you know where he may be hidden?" The Blackbird did not, but wishing to help, led them in turn to all the oldest and most sacred creatures of the forest. The Stag, the Owl and lastly the Eagle were asked in turn, but they too knew not of Mabon.

But the Eagle had sympathy for the weary king and said to him, "In a pool shaded by nine hazel trees, lives the ancient Salmon of Wisdom, even older than I. I can take you to her. The oldest creatures of the land could not tell you where to find Mabon, but perhaps the oldest creature of the water can help."

On arrival at the pool, King Arthur called out, "Salmon of Wisdom! We have come a long way to seek your help. We have spoken to the ancient beings – Blackbird, Stag, Owl, and Eagle – but none could lead us to what we seek. We are looking for Mabon, son of Modron. Do you know where he may be hidden?"

From the depths of the pool, there came a lovely voice like the bubbling of a stream. "The ocean is my home, I know the secrets of its depths – I will take you to Mabon." Quick as light glinting over the water, the Salmon swam carrying Arthur on her back. They approached the place where the stream began its journey, the otherworld, and the spring by the great Castle of Light. Now the Castle of Light was, in fact, dark and overgrown, ruined from long neglect. As the Salmon of Wisdom drew closer, Arthur could hear the weeping from within its stone walls and found the figure of a man huddled in a far corner. At the noise, the man looked up, his face radiant and youthful beneath the streaks of tears. Long had he been locked in these walls.

Arthur said, "I have need of a great huntsman to stalk the wild boar. So, I have come to set you free." Elated, Mabon followed Arthur and the Salmon of Wisdom carried them through splashing waters, and soon all the dirt and strife of that dark time had washed from Mabon's face, and his whole being seemed to shine once again.

His mother swept him up in an embrace of gratitude and happiness. Modron helped Arthur hunt his boar and there followed a great feast and celebration, with Modron and Mabon honoured guests at the King's table.

Blackberries

They [the Fairies] have three great festivals in the year – May Eve, Midsummer Eve, November Eve… On Midsummer Eve, when the bonfires are lighted on every hill in honour of St. John, the fairies are at their gayest [...] on November Eve they are at their gloomiest, for, according to the old Gaelic reckoning, this is the first night of winter. This night they dance with the ghosts, and the pooka* is abroad, and witches make their spells, and girls set a table with food in the name of the devil, that the fetch of their future lover may come through the window and eat of the food. After November Eve the blackberries are no longer wholesome, for the pooka has spoiled them.

William Butler Yeats, *Fairy and Folk Tales of the Irish Peasantry* **(1888)**

---

*   An anglicised variant spelling of *púca* – an irish ghost.

The end of August into September is blackberry season in the British Isles. These wild growing thorny brambles that fill hedgerows and wild spaces, are covered in ripe black berries, free for the taking. They often feature in the harvest feast in a pie or cake or are made into jam.

In English folklore, passing beneath an archway formed by blackberry bramble bushes could cure or prevent a number of ailments, including whooping cough and boils. In Ireland, passing beneath the brambles affords you good luck in card games. There are also protective properties to the plant. Blackberry vines can be woven into wreaths to ward off spirits and witches. But be warned, there is also a legend concerning Lucifer falling into a blackberry bush after being expelled from heaven by St. Michael and spitting on the blackberries to make them bitter so that they cannot be picked after Michaelmas[†] (29th September). In Ireland, it's the púcas that spit on them. And in Scotland, the Devil is said to throw his cloak over the blackberries. Whoever you believe, eating them after Michaelmas is not advised! As is often the case, folklore usually reflects some sensible advice. By early October blackberries are vulnerable to fruit rot, so it really was unwise to eat them, and a few people doing so and getting ill would have been enough to create superstition around it.

Another reason blackberries were not considered good to eat after September was that in October they became witches' food. This may explain a little piece of British blackberry folklore connected to cats, the popular witch familiar: kittens born after the blackberry season ends, were called "Blackberry Kittens," and are thought to be especially mischievous.

Michaelmas and Harvest Festivals in Church

Michaelmas falls on September 29th, and is a Christian quarter day feast. Michaelmas follows the autumn Ember Days, during which Christians traditionally thanked God for his creation and the bounty of the earth and fasted. (There's a lot of alternative feasting and fasting in the Christian calendar.)

The end of the harvest was often celebrated with a big meal called a Harvest Supper, eaten on Michaelmas Day. Traditional feasting food was a goose

---

[†]   Also called St. Michael's Mass, or the Feast day of Michael and All Angels.

stuffed with apples, which was eaten along with a variety of vegetables. Goose fairs were, and still are, held in English towns at this time of year.

Harvest Festivals in churches could be held on the Sunday nearest the Harvest Moon (the full moon that occurs closest to the Autumn Equinox) and often include decorating churches with home-grown fruit and veg, which is then given to those in need.

Autumn Embers

Fasting days and Emberings be
Lent, Whitsun, Holyrood, and Lucie.

***

Lenty, Penty, Crucy, Lucy...
Old English Rhymes for remembering the Ember Days

It is a custom among many Christians to observe Ember Days: clusters of three days in the calendar year, roughly around the start of the four seasons. They are set aside by the Church as a way to mark the passage of seasons and give thanks for nature's gifts through prayer and fasting. Apparently, the name is derived from the Latin *quattuor tempora,* meaning "four times/seasons," but I certainly see whispers of pagan/Celtic fire festivals here.

The Kitchen Witch's Hedgerow and Garden

The morning mists lift slowly now; autumnal sunshine gleams on hedgerows and orchards bursting with crops. The last golden rays of summer have departed to make way for the russets, bronzes and ochres of autumn. Crows caw as they jump through harvested fields. The time of the second harvest is the last gathering of the grain and the fruits that have ripened under the summer sun. In the cauldron, these fruits become syrups, chutneys and jams to stock our winter cupboards.

The forager might spot in the hedgerows: elderberries, damsons, crab apples, and blackberries. The apple trees are bowed with fruit, and oak trees are laden with acorns. Conkers are beginning to peek from their spiny cases. Transition hangs in the air as the light disappears ever earlier each evening.

Kitchen Witch Celebrations for Mabon

It is time to relish and celebrate the harvest whilst readying ourselves, storing what we need and preparing the ground for the winter and the dark to come. The light of the sun in the Wheel of the Year stands in the west, where the sun sets: this is a time of farewell and gratitude for the summer that has been, enjoying the rewards of labour and respect for the land. Mabon, like its opposite on the Wheel, Ostara, is a time of balance. Now, instead of looking to expand outward into summer, we begin drawing inward, preparing ourselves for the winter to come.

Celebrating Today

☽ Gather berries to make wine or steep in gin – damson gin, blackberry wine and elderberry wine are all favourites of mine!

☽ Make elderberry syrup for warding off colds and flu during the long winter months.

☽ Make chutney, juice, cider and cake with the apple crops.

☽ Gather conkers and display in your kitchen – English superstition says they ward off spiders and moths!

☽ Plant spring bulbs – daffodils, snowdrops, bluebells and garlic for next year.

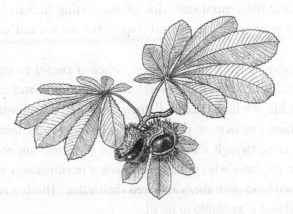

SECTION FOUR SUMMARY

For most of our history, humans had to respect the seasons and pay close attention to cycles such as the moon, season and sun simply as part of survival. Festivals, feast days and holy days, helped people find balance and connection in an uncertain world and, for many, continue to do so in the present, as humanity and the natural environment draw further and further apart. The Wheel, like any tradition, is one of constant change; but continues to be meaningful to many in attuning to the cycles and changes of the year.

While cunning crafts and folk beliefs are diminished in our modern culture, many are still with us, blended into modern cultural practice, like apple bobbing, bonfires, candles on cakes and regional songs of blessing and goodwill. But it may be that many have become almost invisible to us as having connection to older folk magics. It can be easy to forget sometimes how present folklore and practices still are in our day-to-day lives and events.

So many histories have become part of the stories and rituals we have inherited and explored in this section. Those who would be branded as "witch" and "pagan" were carrying rural traditions and ancient customs. The simple celebrations, and value of what they were doing, like utilising local herbs and celebrating the seasons have been clouded by so much hearsay, superstition, and just plain disdain by those who, for centuries, dominated writing, publishing and religious institutions.

Some timeless facets of seasonal festivity have remained in place, including what is probably the central one: that of connecting human beings to the rhythm of the seasons, reverence and respect for the natural world and the weather.

For many modern witches and pagans, when it comes to honouring the sacred, connection to the natural world and community and celebration of the seasons of life, we have come full circle and arrived back where we started: placing these practices at the front and centre of our lives, personally and publicly. Even though these festivals were once relevant to everyone in centuries past, it's those who most keenly seek a reconnection with the land that have helped hold onto them and seen their value. This is a rural past that connects us all and is available to us all.

One might question if modern additions to old traditions negate their authenticity or relevance. But I believe that the reworkings and structures brought by new practitioners and religions allow us to reinvigorate old practices and bring them back into lived experience once more (and as many a tale will remind us, change happens and will continue to happen whether we approve or not).

As always, the witch is ever practical. We have lost so many of the practices and rituals of our ancestors; in some instances, we have had no choice but to create new ones. And isn't this creation, in fact, a beautiful part of the witch's path or any adventure in wayfinding: adding to the living folklore of our cultures? Each festival, each point on the Wheel, has always been an invitation to pause, reflect, offer gratitude, and celebrate. To create cakes that one would offer to everyone from goddess to beggar, enjoy and take hope from the cleansing powers of fire, and offer food to the earth. New ideas and ways are new blossoms on the tree whose roots remain deep in the ancient earth.

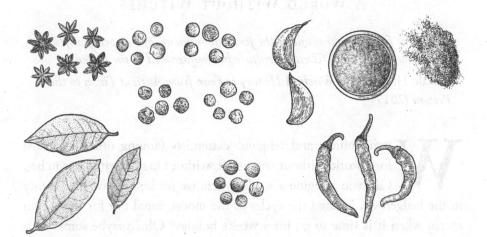

CLOSING

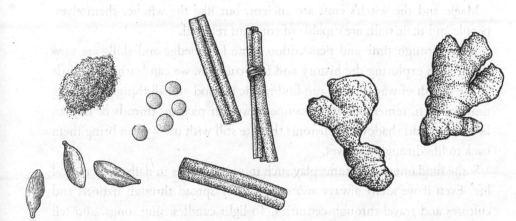

A WORLD WITHOUT WITCHES

The witch figure remains one of the few embodiments of independent female power that traditional Western culture has bequeathed to the present.

Ronald Hutton, *The Witch: A History of Fear, from Ancient Times to the Present* (2017)

Witch hunters and religious extremists (among others) yearned for a world without witchcraft, without magic, without witches. Can you imagine a world where we no longer saw the bounty in the hedgerows, ignored the cycles of the moon, cared not for the season except when it is time to go for a week's holiday? Oh...maybe some of us aren't that far off! And if that sounds like your life, it's not your fault: this is simply a reality of modern living and decades of cultural disconnection from the seasonal practices of our ancestors.

If you want to reclaim your magic, all you need to do is make a start. Perhaps by bringing your awareness to the seasons, the moon, to herbs, to the food you prepare and the stories connected to it...and soon enough you'll remember: this stuff runs in your bones after all.

Perhaps this book has helped you see the value and magic of remembering the food of your ancestors, beloved family members and foods of your childhood; to appreciate the healing and nourishing qualities of herbs and vegetables and the stories connected to them. And remember, as often as you can, to offer gratitude and reverence for the earth: we owe nothing less than our very existence to the soil beneath our feet, and the plants that grow in it.

Magic and the witch's craft are ancient, but like the witches themselves, people and their skills are capable of constant renewal.

Sadly through time and persecution some knowledge and skills are now lost. But in exploring the history and folk customs, we can learn just a little of the wealth of ways people can find magic in food and all things. In taking time to learn, remember and reconnect, we can pick up threads of human behaviours and shadows of customs that are still with us. We can bring them back to life through our lives.

Some fundamental customs play such important roles in daily and cultural life. Even if we aren't always aware of it, they spread through nations and cultures and travel through centuries. To light candles, sing songs, and tell stories, we may have forgotten why we connect in this way, but we can feel its importance once we are sat in circle.

As the wise Professor Hutton says, the witch figure remains with us in the worldwide consciousness: magic, stories, folklore and the witch has continued to be part of our lives despite those who sought to burn them out of existence. Witches survived, and magic survives.

The witch today is different, but every bit as powerful as the figure of ancient times, of witch trials and of fairy tale. The witch figure, now, more than ever, is a muse to creative imagination, ambition, strength, resilience, and encouragement to get better acquainted with yourself and your desires, your place in nature and in the world.

Witches remain because they are important.

NEEDFUL THINGS

Once, magic, rituals, deities were considered to be central to securing our most basic of needs: food, shelter, health, safety and our fear of losing these universal needs. Ritual like that of Ninkasi and her beer seem beautiful to us now, and I'm sure they were then as well; but they were also vital for making something safe to drink: unsafe water could kill whole communities. Safe drinking water, a good harvest…these things weren't a given in the past, so they were prepared and received with much gratitude, ritual and ceremony, celebrated as sacred.

And when the image of the witch swept through centuries, she was feared because she represented a threat to these basic needs: stealing food, putting out hearth fires, spoiling butter, killing cattle and people on an evil whim. She was a threat to survival to those who feared her. And yet to those who trusted her way, she promised life, protection, and healing. She held the power.

For many of us today, our basic needs are met, so now, perhaps, our intentions of ritual and ceremony are a little different, as we are in a different culture and time. We are still, as always, seeking knowledge, meaning and connection to ancestors and the world, but we no longer, for the most part, live in fear of the gods destroying our harvest or displeasing the goddesses of home and hearth. Maybe now our rituals may bring us to other elements still essential to our well-being: mindfulness, love, and creativity. Maybe we are no longer satisfied by a long commute, or a desk job, senseless consumerism, or striving for status, and we find beliefs in other ways of being bubbling to the surface. We desire to explore the philosophical and emotional connections that magic can offer – an openness to a responsive and incredible universe.

In taking up the position of the witch, we can reclaim the knowledge and power of the natural world, and radically renew our relationship with the earth. Many women's stories have been erased from history, but the witch and the goddesses are images that have been mindfully, fiercely held on to and drawn through history: we can see her clearly in cave painting, stone icons, ancient feminine forms, carved words, stories, embroideries and magical charms. It's hard to explain it sometimes in a way that any academic or scholar would recognise, but many see this history and just *know*, instinctively, primally, something of the magic and hope involved with these depictions of feminine power. Something which our culture has hidden, lost, or forgotten. The recovery of this ancient memory of magic and feminine power is an intense personal revelation and a catalyst for many.

WITCHCRAFT TODAY

In the past, they burned us.
Because they thought we were witches.
Just because we knew what to do with herbs outside of the kitchen
Because we know how to dance, how to seduce, how to pray.
Because we moved with the cycles of the moon.
In the past, they burned us alive
Because they knew that we are witches.

Fleassy Malay, "Witches" (2018)

Witch is a word created for the powerful.

Over time, wild stories and superstitions were woven around this idea. So that now witch means a million things. Good and bad. For a long time, it wasn't (and isn't always today) used as a positive term. Quite the opposite. But the power remains. As do we.

Witchcraft is certainly much more attractive now you can be reasonably sure you won't burn for it. We can now name ourselves witches through the luxury of choice and acceptance, rather than have the accusation hurled at us, potentially resulting in torture, ostracisation, and death.

With this increased freedom, we can explore more deeply perhaps who we are and what our values and passions are. We may choose to identify ourselves in line with our interests and passions and use these new terms, should we wish: Green Witch, Hedge Witch…and of course, Kitchen Witch. They are not ancient terms, but new ones to categorise certain skills. They acknowledge that witches, like people, come in many different expressions, with many different interests. They can help us find kindred spirits, extending a web of connection to networks of other witches practising the craft in a similar way, who can become guiding lights and bright mirrors to help us navigate the path of living: as a human and a witch.

These new freedoms and choices encourage an element of play, pushing the boundaries, figuring out what witchcraft can be for us in the modern-day, and looking at what it was and has been through history. And perhaps we recognise now more than ever that we don't have the authority to tell someone else who they are. We don't get to say what magic is for anyone but ourselves. One person does not get to dictate who is a witch and who isn't, what ritual is worthy and what isn't. There are elements of witches' beliefs or magic that will remain unexplained, and we needn't fear that.

Each culture has its own traditional connections to magic, and for some they are a point of reconnection to the magic of the past, as well as a stepping stone to bringing traditional witchcraft into the present and future. The stories of the Kitchen Witch bring us ideas of how to embrace magic today, right now, in an accessible, simple, homespun and practical way.

Claiming the title of Kitchen Witch is not about being stuck in the kitchen, but taking power through it. Along with other realms outside of it. It is about having the freedom to find magic in your daily life and actions. Witches have always crept along the boundaries between peace and chaos, innocence and evil, attraction and aversion, the natural and supernatural. The witch's influence has grown as we have brought them out of the shadows. With this power, we have a choice – which kind of witch do we want to be? What stories do we want to share, or what is the story we want to create?

Moving forward is to perhaps break free of patriarchal methods of attempted destruction, domination and hate, obsessions with a hidden group of enemies. Our challenge is (among other things) to not become what our oppressors were and are, but to do what the divine feminine and the Kitchen Witch do so well: build, nourish and grow. Our task: to see what good can we gather from the broken fragments and forgotten histories. One way, as I've covered in these pages, is through celebration and remembering of food and its glorious folklore and story.

This, like much of my writing, is a personal reclamation of the word witch. And it can be a personal reclamation of yours to see magic, make magic, embody magic. You may not fully be able to reclaim the word witch as a positive…yet. It is, for many of us, the work of a lifetime. But know that there are many, many others walking this path too: reclaiming the heritage and legacy of the witches of the past and bringing her into the present. From feminist writers who first worked to share the words and names of witches, to novelists that feature the beauty of the Kitchen Witch working magic through food. From campaigners working hard to get a new national memorial for the lost lives of many thousands in the Scottish witch trials, to those seeking to create safe communities for practicing witches today. And wonderful projects celebrating the healing powers of the women accused, and the ongoing process of healing from such ancestral trauma like the Medicine Spoon Memorial by artist Caren Thompson.

Friend, there is evil in this world, but perhaps now we understand that we should all be more fearful of the system and the prejudices of those that burnt the witches than the witches themselves.

KITCHEN WITCH AND THE VALUE OF MAGIC

Civilisation began with magic, offerings, rituals, and connection to the natural world – listening, learning, growing. It is the foundation of our species. It has been a rocky path, and it still is for some. But the witch – and her magic – remains in our stories, our superstitions, our empowerment, and our suffering.

I hope you have enjoyed reminding yourself of the magic of food and exploring just some of the unique possibilities and opportunities it offers us. A past that wasn't easier, or even simpler, but that perhaps was better connected to elements of our wellbeing that we are missing now: gratitude for food, sharing food with others, eating seasonally, and seeing the healing power in plants.

Connecting to traditions and customs of times past is not about a wholesale return to the past, but rather connecting to the wisdom and knowledge of our ancestors: recognising its value and bringing that forward into the present.

Food is the most everyday magic – but in the rush of modern life it's easy to forget that it is magic at all. I hope I have made it clear that once you peel away the layers of the storybook magician, the cruel witch on her broomstick, the wise man of the woods who talks to fairies, the pointy hats and fiendish familiars...what you are left with is a simple craft of bringing nourishment and healing to the table, a desire to bring a sense of wonder and enchantment into the kitchen and the food you eat, and a fascination with the stories, symbols and meaning behind it all.

With all magic, there is an element of choice and intention, to see things as completely benign, or to see the potential for magic, is entirely up to you. Witchcraft and magic are only really effective if we believe in them – for better or worse. As Roald Dahl famously told us, "Those who don't believe in magic will never find it."

Magic is everywhere, if we choose to find it: in the connections from the big – the moon, earth, seasons, harvest – to the tiny – a cup of tea, a cinnamon cookie lovingly prepared and eaten joyfully gathered around the hearth fire.

STRONG MEDICINE

Words can be strong medicine. Stories can touch our hearts and souls; they can point the way to healing and transformation.

Our own lives are stories that we write from day to day; they are journeys through the dark of the fairy tale woods.

The tales of previous travellers through the woods are passed down to us in the poetic, symbolic language of folklore and myth; where we step, someone has stepped before, and their stories can help light the way.

Terri Windling, artist and storyteller [23]

To accuse someone of witchcraft was once a curse, but as times change and the world's consciousness grows, it means so much more. Witch is, and always will be, a powerful word, and if we have learnt anything through the pages of this book, it is perhaps that words (and stories) are powerful, "strong medicine" as Terri Windling says. They may light a way for steps on our path or be a spark for change, a cue for necessary breaking down and rebuilding. They can be everything from a gentle warm candle flame to a stick of dynamite.

Standing on the shoulders of our ancestors helps us see further perhaps: they have walked this way before, and although the journey, like a spiral, is different with every cycle, the words of those who knew, and who went before us can help guide our way. I am very grateful for the words of all those who came before, of those who were called witches, as well as those who saw the value of these words and preserved them, passing them down the generations to reach us here. Not all of us can still learn these ancient ways by the hearth fire. But by uncovering the words of witches past, drawing them back into the light, we can learn, we can mourn, we can celebrate, and we can grow. We can write our own magical folklore – in story, in food, in the paths we walk.

Some things don't change...and maybe that's why food can be so comforting. In an ever-changing world, a hot drink will always be warming to body and soul; a meal with friends will always be comforting; eating your family's favourite food will always remind you of them. When you are hungry and tired, supper waiting for you when you get home will always be a treat.

But many things do change... We have seen over centuries that faith in magic has waned. We have watched through history "The gradual transformation of the gods into devils, of the wise women into witches, of the worship into superstitious customs" (Grimm, *Deutsche Mythologie*) and pagan festivals and customs transformed into Christian ones. But fear not, if you look, magic is still here. Goddesses and witches hide as saints. And the names of the deities have found hiding places in months and years, names of our foods, plants and spices: goddesses Artemis, Iris, and Hebe still live in our world, and our gardens. The lore of the land is kept alive in the whispers of grasses in the wind: to some ragwort is still called the Fairies' Horse, along with Elf Grass and The Fairy Flax (wild grasses). We have Witches' Butter (fungi), Witches' Bells (bluebells) and Witches' Thimbles (foxgloves). Scraps of magical and pagan practices are still running through the seams of our language, customs and history, not least through our stories, and so sharing them is essential in keeping ideas alive that which could be lost.

Luckily, our roots as farmers and people of the land run deep, and intuitive connections still exist. Quieter now, perhaps, it can take a little work to hear the call of the wild places and the green spaces. But slowly, quietly, more and more of us feel a desire to return to natural rhythms and cycles. And our relationships with plants, land and food are blooming once again: the spirits of the witches, healers and herbwives of days past watch over the chefs, nutritionists, and herbalists of today.

Your Own Coven

This book is the longest I have ever written, and yet, I have barely scratched the surface of the wealth of stories surrounding food folklore and the witches that dance through the tales and superstitions. There was so much more I could have included. My hope is that I have both retold some of your favourites, as well as offering you tastes of new stories and characters and wisdom. Food is a topic that is both shared, and yet is so personal to each and every one of us on this planet. We all have our own stories of food, of coming together, the food that makes us feel better and that evokes memories. So, should you feel that your favourite food or fairy tale is missing from this book, I advise you to seek your coven: your mothers, aunts, cousins, siblings, peers, friends, elders and wise ones and retell your stories together, make your family foods together, write down the recipes and stories, share them with others.

Your Own Hearth

I hope that meeting the Kitchen Witch, exploring the magic of folklore and superstitions has helped you reconnect to the magic of food, its stories and the magic of your own cultures and heritage. I personally have learnt so much about the origins of magic, witchcraft and the knowledge of the witches through researching and writing it.

When it comes to food, the kitchen, magic and witchcraft, nothing is really new. So, when you bake your bread, gather your herbs, brew your infusions, remember…well, just remember. Let the magic of memory and ancestry lay its hand gently on your shoulder as you cook.

Thank you for joining me, witches and wise ones.

"Beer, Cakes, Meat…Drink, Dance, and Have Music…
Merry meet, Merry part."[24]

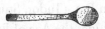

GLOSSARY AND TIMELINE

PEOPLE AND AGES OF THE BRITISH ISLES AND EUROPE

The British Isles are a mix of Celtic, Anglo-Saxon, Roman, and Viking/Norse cultures. So, we have an amazing collection of monuments, artefacts, deities, stories and folklore from ancient Celtic, pagan, Christian, Norse, Roman, and Germanic beliefs (as well as our most recent native religion, Wicca).

In order to bring some of what I have said into context it seems important to include a very rough outline. So, using the Encyclopaedia Britannica as my touchstone, this is a rough outline of five main historical eras: Ancient History, Classical, Middle Ages, Early Modern, and Modern eras. (You will see these dates vary wildly from sources and for difference places.)

Ancient History The Stone Age began about 2.6 million years ago, and lasted until the Bronze Age began. Being such a long period, it's divided into three respective periods: the Palaeolithic, Mesolithic and the Neolithic. What we consider to be modern humans, Homo sapiens, appear in the Palaeolithic period.

2500 BCE The Bronze Age.

1000 BCE The Iron Age which lasts up to the Roman invasion of Britain.

43 CE to 410 CE. Roman Britain. Followed by a short period of time where the Germanic tribes that we could collectively call the Anglo-Saxons begin to arrive in Britain.

500 to 1400/1500 CE The Middle Ages, also known as Medieval, and I have used them interchangeably throughout the book. (Viking invasions came and went in this era, the Anglo-Saxon era ended too. And this was also the beginning of many centuries of European witch hunts.)

1500-1837 The Early Modern Era. (Tudor, Stuart and Georgian periods respectively, this period also includes the Age of Enlightenment and the rise of modern science, and saw the official end to the European witch hunts.)

1837-1914 Victorian and Edwardian eras, times of massive industrialisation and urbanisation in England and the expansion of Empire.

Modern Era The 1900s and beyond.

PEOPLE

Celts and Gaels: Celt is a term applied to a group of Iron Age tribes spread across Europe and the British Isles from their homeland in south-central Europe from around 1200 BCE. It was the ancient Greeks who created the word Celt, using it to refer to anyone in Europe north of the Mediterranean. From the word *keltoi* (meaning barbarian).

There are a variety of languages/groups that live under the Celtic umbrella: including Gaelic (Irish and Scottish versions), Cornish, Welsh, Manx, Briton and Breton.

Scotland, Ireland, and the Isle of Man are allied as Gaelic, joined together by common Gaelic language and cultures, and natives may refer to themselves as Gaels. With invasions of the Romans and the Germanic tribes, Celts got pushed out to the edges of Britain, so now when we think of Celts, it's the native languages and culture in Ireland, Scotland, the Isle of Man, Wales, Cornwall and a little of northern France. Celtic tradition was primarily verbal, so there's little documentation of the culture, but artefacts, carvings and burial sites offer us clues.

Druids: Members of the learned class among the ancient Celts, often priests and teachers. The earliest known records of the Druids come from 300 BCE. Their name has various etymological connections to the oak tree, so translations usually come up as 'knower of the oak' or 'oak seer.'

Anglo-Saxon: The Anglo-Saxons were members of the Germanic peoples from areas we know today as Denmark, Netherlands and Northern Germany; people known as the Angles, the Saxons and the Jutes all came together to form the Anglo-Saxons. They settled in territories that are today part of England and Wales, from the end of Roman rule up to 1066. We would describe these tribes as mainly pagan and they followed a Germanic pantheon of gods similar to beliefs that ran through Scandinavia.

Pagan: The term paganus is a derivative of the Latin word *pagus,* meaning "rustic", so those fancy-pants city dwellers might refer to someone who lives in the countryside as paganus! The term pagan later became associated with someone who followed ancient, primal, pre-Christian religions. It was often used to refer to anyone who believed in a pantheon of gods rather than one God. Witchcraft and paganism are often linked together as many witchcraft practices draw from pagan practices and vice versa. Heathen originally referred to Germanic paganism: the Heathens were the pre-Christian Northern European peoples, including in Anglo-Saxon England, Scandinavia and Germany. People from Celtic roots may self-identify as pagan. Whereas those who follow more Germanic/Norse may refer to themselves as "heathen," which, like pagan, is connected to country-folk meaning "heath dweller."

Wicca: A religion native to England created around the 1940s and 50s. Followers of this religion call themselves witches. The word "wicca" is from Old English roots and meaning "to weave/bend", and was later used to refer to a witch or worker of magic. There are, however, like lots of religions, many splinter Wiccan groups all over the world: Gardnerian Wicca, Alexandrian Wicca, Dianic Wicca – with many conflicting and contrasting views.

To be a witch and/or practise magic is ancient. Wicca as a religion is much more modern. But you may also come across witches that are so named for their following of the Wiccan religion. And Wiccan practices are often drawn from older witchcraft practices. Pagan and witch are not necessarily the same thing, although they overlap: and you can be both. Paganism is a complex of religions, old and new, that centre on deities of pre-Christian Europe. A pagan that practises magic may also call themselves a witch.

COVEN OF CONTRIBUTORS

A huge thank you to my triple goddesses: Mercedes, Khyati and Alexis for sharing their words and enriching my book!

Mercedes Reyes is the CEO and founder of Bruja Coffee Co. Based in New Mexico, specialising in organic small batch artisan coffee, ceremonial cacao, and medicinal teas. She uses traditional roasting practices from her native lands and is gifted in her craft of making the coffee experience a magical one.

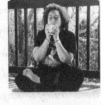

bruja-coffee-co.myshopify.com

Khyati Patel is an aspiring Clinical Psychologist, currently working as a Psychological Wellbeing practitioner, she is interested in all that is related to mental health. Her love for food comes from growing up eating delicious generational recipes cooked by her mum and maternal grandmother to help her feel more connected to her Indian roots whilst growing up in London. Khyati firmly believes that food is the magic that connects all around the table.

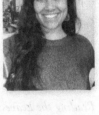

Alexis Prior is a BANT and CNHC Registered Nutritional Therapist who works with busy women over forty as they transition through midlife and perimenopausal health changes. She follows the functional medicine approach, which means her clients get a personalised, detailed investigation into their health issues and a plan that works for them to help them get their oomph back.

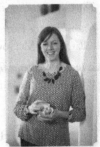

alexispriornutrition.com

And special thanks to *Independent Spirit of Bath,* Bath's finest purveyors of whisky and many libations, who helped me bring the stories of the alewives and the angel's share to life.

BIBLIOGRAPHY

FOODWAYS AND FOLKLORE

The Magic Harvest: Food, Folklore and Society – Piero Camporesi

The Hearth Witch's Compendium – Anna Franklin

A Hedgerow Cookbook – Glennie Kindred

Folklore and Odysseys of Food and Medicinal Plants – Ernst and Johanna Lehner

The Food and Folklore reader: Collected Academic Essays – Lucy M. Long (ed.)

The Magick of Food: Rituals, Offerings and Why We Eat Together – Gwion Raven

Good Things in England: A Practical Cookery Book for Everyday Use – Florence White

DRINKS

Ale, Beer and Brewsters in England: Women's Work in a Changing World, 1300-1600 – Judith M. Bennett

Café Nation: Coffee Folklore, Magick and Divination – Sandra Mizumoto Posey

Whisky Legends of Islay – Robin Laing

The Whisky Muse: Scotch Whisky in Poem and Song – Robin Laing

Peat Smoke and Spirit: The Story of Islay and its Whiskies – Andrew Jefford

Reading the Leaves: An Intuitive Guide to the Ancient Art and Modern Magic of Tea Leaf Divination – Sandra Maria Wright and Leanne Marrama

Tea-Cup Reading and Fortune-Telling by Tea Leaves – A Highland Seer (1881)

Uncorking the Past: The Quest for Wine, Beer, and Other Alcoholic Beverages (First Edition) – Patrick E. McGovern

Whiskey Women: The Untold Story of How Women Saved Bourbon, Scotch, and Irish Whiskey – Fred Minnick

THE WITCH AND NOTABLE WOMEN

The Witch in History: Early Modern and Twentieth-Century Representations – Diane Purkiss

The Witchcraft Reader – Darren Oldridge (ed.)

Witches and Pagans: Women in European Folk Religion, 700-1100 – Max Dashu

Hildegard of Bingen: The Woman of Her Age – Fiona Maddocks

The Witch: A History of Fear, from Ancient Times to the Present – Ronald Hutton

Witches, Druids and King Arthur – Ronald Hutton

Witches, Midwives, and Nurses: A History of Women Healers
– Deirdre English and Barbara Ehrenreich

Witch Hunt – Kristen J. Sollee

The Encyclopaedia of Witches and Witchcraft – Rosemary Guiley

Woman, Church and State – Matilda Joslyn Gage

Daughters of Hecate: Women and Magic in the Ancient World
– Kimberly B. Stratton and Dayna S. Kalleres

Yoga for Witches – Sarah Robinson

Burning Woman – Lucy H. Pearce

The Witchcraft Sourcebook – Brian P. Levack (ed.)

Borders Witch Hunt: The Story of the 17th Century Witchcraft Trials in the Scottish Borders
– Mary W. Craig

HERBALS

Culpeper's Complete Herbal – Nicholas Culpeper

The Herball or Generall Historie of Plantes – John Gerard (also spelt Gerarde and often known today in modern printings as *Gerard's Herbal*)

The Old English Herbals – Eleanour Sinclair Rohde

Gattefosse's Aromatherapy – Rene Gattefosse

ANCIENT GREECE AND ROME

Women and Power: A Manifesto – Professor Mary Beard

SPQR: A History of Ancient Rome – Professor Mary Beard

Arcana Mundi: Magic and the Occult in Greek and Roman World – George Luck

ANCIENT, ANGLO-SAXON AND MEDIEVAL TEXTS (VIEWED ONLINE VIA ARCHIVES/DATABASES)

The Anglo-Saxon Chronicles (translations can be found online at gutenberg.org and archive.org)

Lacnunga, Bald's Leechbook and *The Reckoning of Time* by Bede (can be viewed at the British Library or via their online catalogue: www.bl.uk)

The Ulster Cycle body of medieval Irish heroic legends and sagas including the *Tochmarc Emire* – The Wooing of Emer (can be found at: celt.ucc.ie)

The Mabinogion – within which is the collection of tales known as *The Mabinogi* (can be found en.wikisource.org/wiki/The_Mabinogion)

Kalevala: the Epic Poem of Finland – Elias Lönnrot (can be found online at gutenberg.org)

FAIRY TALES AND FOLKLORE

Fairy Tales (Les Contes des Fées) – Marie-Catherine d'Aulnoy (1697) as translated by Annie Macdonell and Miss Lee, (1892)

Tales and Stories of the Past with Morals or Tales of Mother Goose (Histoires ou Contes du Temps Passé or Contes de ma Mère l'Oye) – Charles Perrault (new translation by Charles Welsh in 1901)

Household tales with other traditional remains, collected in The Counties of York, Lincoln, Derby, and Nottingham – Sidney Oldall Addy (1895)

Wenn Die Fusche Kaffee Kochen (When the Foxes Make Coffee) – Angela Sommer-Bodenburg

The Wisdom of Fairy Tales – Rudolf Meyer

The Original Folk and Fairy Tales of the Brothers Grimm: The Complete First Edition – Jack Zipes (trans.)

Kinder und Hausmärchen (Children's and Household Tales) – Jacob and Wilhelm Grimm 1812-1815 (Volumes 1 and 2)

English Fairy Tales – Flora Annie Steel

Russian Wonder Tales – Post Wheeler

Gypsy Sorcery and Fortune Telling – Charles Godfrey Leland (1891)

The Celtic Twilight – W. B. Yeats

Irish Fairy Tales – James Stephens

Russian Fairy Tales: A Choice Collection of Muscovite Folk-lore – W. R. S. Ralston

English Fairy Tales – Joseph Jacobs

The Fairy-Faith in Celtic Countries – W. Y. Evans-Wentz

Witchcraft and Superstitious Record in the South-Western District of Scotland
The Folklore of Orkney and Shetland – Ernest Marwick

Northern Mythology – Benjamin Thorpe (1852)

Scottish Customs – Sheila Livingstone

Fairy and Folk Tales of the Irish Peasantry – William Butler Yeats (1888)

Irish Witchcraft and Demonology – St. John D. Seymour

Cornish Saints and Sinners – J. Henry Harris (1906)

Cornish Feasts and Folk-lore – M. A. Courtney

Traditions, Superstitions and Folk-lore – Charles Hardwick (1872)

From Three Goddesses: Walburg, Verena and Gertrud as German Church Saints – E.L. Rochholz, (1870) (translated from German)

The Mysteries of All Nations: Strange Customs Fables and Tales – James Grant (1880)

Demonology and Devil-lore – Moncure Daniel Conway

Letters on Demonology and Witchcraft – Walter Scott

Folk-Lore of West and Mid-Wales – Jonathan Ceredig Davies

Celtic Mythology and Religion – Alexander Macbain

A Handbook of Saxon Sorcery and Magic – Alaric Albertsson

Deutsche Mythologie (Teutonic Mythology)
– Jacob Grimm. Translated by James Steven Stallybrass

Celtic Folklore: Welsh and Manx (Volumes 1+2) – John Rhys

Plant Lore, Legends, and Lyrics – Richard Folkard

Folk-Lore of West and Mid-Wales – Jonathan Ceredig Davies

A Tour in Scotland – Thomas Pennant (1769)

Russian Fairy Tales – Moura Budberg and Amabel Williams-Ellis

Dancing at Lughnasa – Brian Friel

Witch-Hunting Texts and Pamphlets

Malleus Maleficarum – Heinrich Kramer (1487)
I used the 1928 English translation by Montague Summers

Formicarius – Johannes Nider (1475)

Fortalitium Fidei – Alphonso de Espina (1485)

The Discovery of Witches – Matthew Hopkins (1647)

The Discoverie of Witchcraft – Reginald Scot (1584)

Saducismus Triumphatus – Joseph Glanvill (1681)

Daemonologie – King James I (known as King James VI in Scotland) (1597)

The Confessions of the Forfar Witches – Joseph Anderson (1661)

Witch Stories – E. Lynn Linton (1861)

The Wonderful Discoverie of the Witchcrafts of Margaret and Philip Flower (1619)

Wicca, Paganism and the Kitchen Witch

Cunningham's Encyclopaedia of Magical Herbs and Magic in Food – Scott Cunningham

A Kitchen Witch's Cookbook – Patricia Telesco

La Sorcière – Jules Michelet

The Golden Bough – George James Frazer

Witchcraft Today – Gerald Gardner

Witchcraft for Tomorrow – Doreen Valiente

The Witch-cult in Western Europe: A Study in Anthropology – Margaret Alice Murray

Magic and Witchcraft – George Moir

Ancient Ways: Reclaiming the Pagan Tradition – Pauline Campanelli and Dan Campanelli

Alchemy of Herbs: Transform Everyday Ingredients into Foods and Remedies That Heal
– Rosalee de la Foret

The Witch's Cauldron: The Craft, Lore and Magick of Ritual Vessels
– Laura Tempest Zakroff

The Mystic Cookfire: The Sacred Art of Creating Food to Nurture Friends and Family
– Veronika Sophia Robinson

To Ride a Silver Broomstick – Silver Ravenwolf

True Magick: A Beginner's Guide – Amber K.

Kitchen Witch's World of Magical Herbs and Plants – Rachel Patterson

Kitchen Witchcraft: Crafts of a Kitchen Witch – Rachel Patterson

Modern Magic – Maximilian Schele de Vere (1873)

A Spell in the Wild – Alice Tarbuck

MODERN FICTION

Chocolat – Joanne Harris

Like Water for Chocolate – Laura Esquival

Mistress of the Spices – Chitra Divakaruni

Half Spent was the Night – Ami McKay

Practical Magic – Alice Hoffman

Hallowe'en Party – Agatha Christie

The Discovery of Chocolate – James Runcie

FESTIVE AND SEASONAL CELEBRATIONS

A Right Merrie Christmas: The Story of Christ-tide – John Ashton (1894)

The Stations of the Sun: A History of the Ritual Year in Britain – Ronald Hutton

The Magical Year: Seasonal Celebrations to Honour Nature's Ever-Turning Wheel
– Danu Forest

History of Christmas Food and Feasts – Claire Hopley

The Old Magic of Christmas: Yuletide Traditions for the Darkest Days of the Year
– Linda Raedisch

The Festival of Lughnasa – Maire MacNeill

A Christmas Cornucopica – Mark Forsyth

The Book of Hallowe'en – Ruth Edna Kelley

Christmas in Ritual and Tradition, Christian and Pagan – Clement A. Miles

The Cassell Dictionary of Folklore – David Pickering

Essays/Articles

"Woman as Witch" – Karl Pearson (1897)

"Kitchen Essays" – Agnes Jekyll (1922)

"Kitchen Witch" – Alice Tarbuck, dangerouswomenproject.org

"Legacies: Old Ways in the Shadow of the Witch Hunts" – Max Dashu

"Magic and animism in old religions: the relevance of sun cults in the world-view of traditional societies" – Georg W. Oesterdiekhoff

"The Celtic Calendar and the Anglo-Saxon Year" – Richard Sermon

"From Easter to Ostara: the reinvention of a pagan goddess?" – Richard Sermon

"Witches, wives and mothers: witchcraft persecution and women's confessions in seventeenth-century England" – Louise Jackson

"A Hymn to Ninkasi"
– J. Dyneley Prince *The American Journal of Semitic Languages and Literatures* Vol. 33

"Brigit: Goddess, Saint, 'Holy Woman', and Bone of Contention" – Carole M Cusack

"Ergotism: The Satan Loosed in Salem? Convulsive ergotism may have been a physiological basis for the Salem witchcraft crisis in 1692"
– Linnda R. Caporael from *Science* Vol. 192 (April 1976)

"About Naming Ostara, Litha and Mabon", Aidan Kelly, Patheos.com (2017)

Miscellaneous

Letters of John Keats to His Family and Friends Sidney Colvin (ed.)

Francis Bacon, Of the Commission of Sales. Apothegms, New and Old – (1625)

The British Housewife or the cook, housekeeper's and gardener's companion – Martha Bradley (1756)

A Sailor of King George, the journals of captain Frederick Hoffman, 1793–1814

The Prairie Light Review; Vol. 9 ; No. 2 , Article 50. (Deborah Joyce Poem "Pasta")

Sacred Home: Creating Shelter for Your Soul – Laurine Morrison Meyer

The Story of My Life – Ellen Terry

A History of the Cries of London – Charles Hindley

Faust: A Tragedy – Johann Wolfgang von Goethe

The Mousehole Cat – Antonia Barber

ONLINE SOURCES

Many of the older books were found on projectgutenburg.com, archive.org, bl.uk and openlibrary.org

worldhistory.org

britannica.com

womeninantiquity.wordpress.com

historycollection.com

suppressedhistories.net

witchesofscotland.com

treespiritwisdom.com

irishwildflowers.ie

Danielle Prohom Olson – gathervictoria.com

Terri Windling – terriwindling.com

Fleassy Malay – fleassymalay.com – "Witches"

Survey of Scottish Witchcraft Database – witches.shca.ed.ac.uk

John Crogintons will 1599 mentioning the 'witche in the kytchyn' – websfor.me.uk/crudgington/wills/john1599_will.asp

The Nine Herbs Charm

herbalhistory.org

wyrtig.com

Hymn to Ninkasi

Oxford University Sumerian literature database – etcsl.orinst.ox.ac.uk

Yale University Babylonian Archives – babylonian-collection.yale.edu

Library of fairy and folk tales compiled by DL Ashliman at University of Pittsburgh – pitt.edu/~dash/folktexts.html

Plus

The story of Arima the Milan Witch was discovered in the gorgeous travel documentary series *Searching for Italy* with Stanley Tucci.

ENDNOTES

1 First said by Harvard professor Laurel Thatcher Ulrich and requoted by many.

2 Titus Livius, Roman historian.

3 From John Crogintons' 1599 will – found at: websfor.me.uk/crudgington under 'wills'. In later generations the surname becomes Crudgington.

4 *The Discoverie of Witchcraft* (1584)

5 *The Discoverie of Witchcraft* (1584)

6 Maximilian Schele de Vere – *Modern Magic* (1873)

7 Ernest Marwick – *The Folklore of Orkney and Shetland* (1975)

8 Richard Folkard – *Plant Lore, Legends, and Lyrics* (1884), *The Oxford Handbook of Witchcraft in Early Modern Europe and Colonial America* edited by Brian P. Levack (2013)

9 Michael Castleman – *The New Healing Herbs* (2017)

10 Emily Gerard – *The Land Beyond the Forest: Facts, Figures, and Fancies from Transylvania* (1888)

11 Linnda R. Caporael – "Ergotism: The Satan Loosed in Salem? Convulsive ergotism may have been a physiological basis for the Salem witchcraft crisis in 1692" *Science* Vol. 192 (April 1976)

12 Fred Minnick – *Whiskey Women: The Untold Story of How Women Saved Bourbon, Scotch, and Irish Whiskey* (2013)

13 Scott Cunningham – *Magic in Food,* 1990, the title has since been changed to *Wicca in the Kitchen*

14 As told by Richard Folkard in *Plant Lore, Legends, and Lyrics* (1884)

15 Harry Sanabria – *The Anthropology of Latin America and the Caribbean* (2007)

16 moontimechocolate.co.uk and bruja-coffee-co.myshopify.com

17 Martha Few – *Women Who Live Evil Lives: Gender, Religion, and the Politics of Power in Colonial Guatemala* and "Chocolate, Sex and Disorderly Women in late-seventeenth- and early-eighteenth-century Guatemala."

18 Kasper S, et al. "Lavender oil preparation Silexan is effective in generalized anxiety disorder – a randomized, double-blind comparison to placebo and paroxetine." *International Journal of Neuropsychopharmacology* (2014)
    Woelk H, et al. "A multi-center, double-blind, randomised study of the lavender oil preparation Silexan in comparison to Lorazepam for generalized anxiety disorder." *Phytomedicine* (2010)
    Sasannejad P, et al. "Lavender Essential Oil in the Treatment of Migraine Headache: A Placebo-Controlled Clinical Trial." *European Neurology* (2012), Vol.67

19 Brothers Grimm – *Children's and Household Tales* (1812)

20 As told to me by Lucy H. Pearce, author and resident of County Cork.

21 Bede – *The Reckoning of Time* (725)

22 As noted by John Gregorson Campbell in *Superstitions of the Highlands and Islands of Scotland*

23 From terriwindling.com, blog post: "Stories are Medicine."

24 From testimony attributed to Alice Duke, accused witch in the Somerset witch trials, 1664, tweaked ever so slightly for effect. The quote as it appears in Joseph Glanvill's book can be found earlier in this book, amongst the apple folklore of Section Two.

ABOUT THE AUTHOR

S arah Robinson is a yoga teacher and author based in in Bath, UK (once named after a goddess: the ancient Roman town of *Aquae Sulis*). Her background is in science; she holds an MSc Psychology & Neuroscience and has studied at Bath, Exeter and Harvard University. She loves exploring the power of myth, magic and story in both her writing and yoga teaching, and is passionate about helping everyone connect to their own special magic and inner power.

She has two books published previously by Womancraft Publishing; *Yoga for Witches* and *Yin Magic*.

Find Sarah online:
  Website: sentiayoga.com
  Instagram: @Yogaforwitches

INDEX

ABOUT THE ARTIST

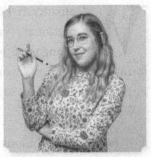

Jessica Roux is a Nashville-based freelance illustrator and plant and animal enthusiast. She loves exploring in her own backyard and being surrounded by an abundance of nature. Using subdued colours and rhythmic shapes, she renders flora and fauna with intricate detail reminiscent of old world beauty.

Find Jessica online:
  Website: jessica-roux.com/
  Instagram: @jessicasroux

ABOUT WOMANCRAFT

Womancraft Publishing was founded on the revolutionary vision that women and words can change the world. We act as midwife to transformational women's words that have the power to challenge inspire, heal and speak to the silenced aspects of ourselves.

We believe that:

(books are a fabulous way of transmitting powerful transformation,

(values should be juicy actions, lived out,

(ethical business is a key way to contribute to conscious change.

At the heart of our Womancraft philosophy is fairness and integrity. Creatives and women have always been underpaid. Not on our watch! We split royalties 50:50 with our authors. We work on a full circle model of giving and receiving: reaching backwards, supporting TreeSisters' reforestation projects, and forwards via Worldreader, providing books at no cost to education projects for girls and women.

We are proud that Womancraft is walking its talk and engaging so many women each year via our books and online. Join the revolution! Sign up to the mailing list at womancraftpublishing.com and find us on social media for exclusive offers:

(f)   womancraftpublishing

(y)   womancraftbooks

(◎)   womancraft_publishing

**Signed copies of all titles available from
shop.womancraftpublishing.com**

THE KITCHEN WITCH COMPANION

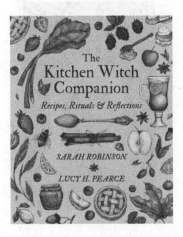

Sarah Robinson & Lucy H. Pearce

The Kitchen Witch returns in this beautifully illustrated companion book to Sarah Robinson's bestseller *Kitchen Witch: Food, Folklore & Fairy Tale*...including many of the traditional and seasonal recipes referenced in that book.

Best-selling authors Sarah Robinson of *Kitchen Witch, Enchanted Journeys, Yoga for Witches* and *Yin Magic* and Lucy H. Pearce of *Burning Woman, Creatrix* and *Medicine Woman* combine forces with a diverse international coven of kitchen witches to share their favourite recipes, rituals and reflections on the magic that can be found...and made in the kitchen.

This is a book to be read curled up in a comfy chair, before being covered in earth as you gather in seasonal goodness and splattered with sauce as you cook! The first half of *The Kitchen Witch Companion* is a nuanced reflection on the fantasy and reality of making magic in the kitchen. The second half is a seasonal collection of recipes and crafts, foraging and ferments, spells and simmer pots, meditations and blessings to inspire you to create, celebrate and gather throughout the Wheel of the Year.

YOGA FOR WITCHES

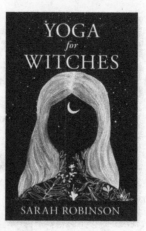

Sarah Robinson

Yoga for Witches explores a new kind of journey, connecting two powerful spiritual disciplines, with enchanting effects! Witchcraft and yoga share many similarities that are explored in combination, in this groundbreaking new title from Sarah Robinson, certified yoga instructor and experienced witch.

Yoga for Witches shares exercises, poses and the knowledge you need to connect to your own special magic and inner power.

☾ Explore how ancient yogis sought out magic.

☾ Weave magic through spells, mantra, meditation and yoga practice.

☾ Discover some of the goddesses and gods of yogic and witch culture.

☾ Connect to the power of the sun, moon and earth via witchcraft and yoga.

☾ Explore the magic of the chakras.

Namaste, Witches!

YIN MAGIC

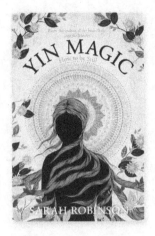

Sarah Robinson

Yin Magic: How to be Still shows how ancient Chinese Taoist alchemical practices can mingle with yoga and magic to enhance our wellbeing from sleep to stress-levels, helping us to move beyond burnout cycles and embody the beauty of letting go. It shares:

☾ What yin is…and why it matters.

☾ An introduction to the practice of yin yoga

☾ Yin yoga journeys for each season and the meridians.

☾ Insight from cutting-edge neuroscience research.

☾ Connections between Celtic, witch and Chinese medicine traditions.

☾ Sympathetic magic and how to bring it into your yoga practice.

☾ How to embrace the magic in the darker times of night, new moon and winter.

Yin Magic helps us to make everyday magic at a sumptuously slow pace as an antidote to the busyness of modern life.

BURNING WOMAN

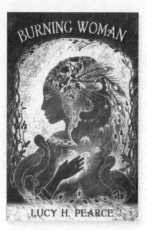

Lucy H. Pearce

Burning Woman is a breath-taking and controversial woman's journey through history – personal and cultural – on a quest to find and free her own power.

Uncompromising and all-encompassing, Lucy H. Pearce uncovers the archetype of the Burning Women of days gone by – Joan of Arc and the witch trials, through to the way women are burned today in cyber bullying, acid attacks, shaming and burnout, fearlessly examining the roots of Feminine power – what it is, how it has been controlled, and why it needs to be unleashed on the world during our modern Burning Times.

Burning Woman explores:

☾ Burning from within: a woman's power – how to build it, engage it and not be destroyed by it.

☾ Burning from without: the role of shame, and honour in the time-worn ways the dominant culture uses fire to control the Feminine.

☾ The darkness: overcoming our fear of the dark, and discovering its importance in cultivating power.

This incendiary text was written for women who burn with passion, have been burned with shame, and who at another time, in another place, would have been burned at the stake. With contributions from leading burning women of our era: Isabel Abbott, ALisa Starkweather, Shiloh Sophia McCloud, Molly Remer, Julie Daley, Bethany Webster ...

USE OF WOMANCRAFT WORK

Often women contact us asking if and how they may use our work. We love seeing our work out in the world. We love you sharing our words further. And we ask that you respect our hard work by acknowledging the source of the words.

We are delighted for short quotes from our books – up to 200 words – to be shared as memes or in your own articles or books, provided they are clearly accompanied by the author's name and the book's title.

We are also very happy for the materials in our books to be shared amongst women's communities: to be studied by book groups, discussed in classes, read from in ceremony, quoted on social media…with the following provisos:

☾ If content from the book is shared in written or spoken form, the book's author and title must be referenced clearly.

☾ The only person fully qualified to teach the material from any of our titles is the author of the book itself. There are no accredited teachers of this work. Please do not make claims of this sort.

☾ If you are creating a course devoted to the content of one of our books, its title and author must be clearly acknowledged on all promotional material (posters, websites, social media posts).

☾ The book's cover may be used in promotional materials or social media posts. The cover art is copyright of the artist and has been licensed exclusively for this book. Any element of the book's cover or font may not be used in branding your own marketing materials when teaching the content of the book, or content very similar to the original book.

☾ No more than two double page spreads, or four single pages of any book may be photocopied as teaching materials.

We are delighted to offer a 20% discount of over five copies going to one address. You can order these on our webshop, or email us. If you require further clarification, email us at: info@womancraftpublishing.com